P9-DXC-525

VEGETABLE JUICING FOR EVERYONE

How to Get Your Family Healthier and Happier, Faster!

Andrew W. Saul, Ph.D.
and Helen Saul Case

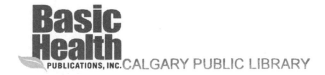

Basic
Health
PUBLICATIONS, INC.

CALGARY PUBLIC LIBRARY

DEC - 2013

And Now a Word from our Sponsor . . . NOT!
We have no financial connection whatsoever with any company in the health products industry. We do not market our own products, nor do we market anyone else's. We do not make
a dime from the sale of juicers, or vitamins, or foods. Or garden seed. Or shovels. We have
no vested interests except our health, your health . . . and you buying armloads of our books
to give to your family and friends. We personally prefer books without product endorse-
ments, and endeavor to offer you the same courtesy.

The information contained in this book is based upon the research and personal and professional experiences of the authors. It is not intended as a substitute for consulting with
your physician or other healthcare provider. Any attempt to diagnose and treat an illness
should be done under the direction of a healthcare professional.

The publisher does not advocate the use of any particular healthcare protocol but believes
the information in this book should be available to the public. The publisher and authors
are not responsible for any adverse effects or consequences resulting from the use of the suggestions, preparations, or procedures discussed in this book. Should the reader have any
questions concerning the appropriateness of any procedures or preparation mentioned, the
authors and the publisher strongly suggest consulting a professional healthcare advisor.

Basic Health Publications, Inc.
28812 Top of the World Drive
Laguna Beach, CA 92651
949-715-7327 • www.basichealthpub.com

Library of Congress Cataloging-in-Publication Data is available
through the Library of Congress.

ISBN 978–1–59120–250–0

Copyright © 2013 by Andrew W. Saul and Helen Saul Case

All rights reserved. No part of this book may be reproduced,
stored in a retrieval system, or transmitted by any means,
electronic, mechanical, photocopying, recording, or otherwise, without written permission from the author.

Editor: Cheryl Hirsch
Typesetting/Book design: Gary A. Rosenberg
Cover design: Mike Stromberg

Printed in the United States of America

10   9   8   7   6   5   4   3   2   1

CONTENTS

To all those who can drink a pint of carrot juice in four seconds flat. And to Dr. Max Gerson, Charlotte Gerson, Norman W. Walker, Paul Bragg, Christopher Gian-Cursio, Jack LaLanne, Dick Gregory, Clara Barton, Bernarr Macfadden, James Caleb Jackson, and all the great natural health crusaders who made us into unashamed health nuts. After all, if you are not a health nut, then what kind of a nut would you rather be?

ACKNOWLEDGMENTS

We would like to thank Charlotte Gerson, Howard Straus, Norm Lee, Nancy Desjardins, Richard Bennett, and John I. Mosher for their great examples and contributions to this project. Our thanks are also extended to the editors of and contributors to the *Orthomolecular Medicine News Service* and the *Journal of Orthomolecular Medicine*.

Special, indeed lavish, appreciation is offered to our very significant others.

And to comedian Victor Borge (1909–2000) who said, "When, once in a while, a handkerchief comes out to wipe away a tear from laughter, that is my reward. The rest goes to the government." You just know a book is going to be a bit off-center when the authors make jokes in the Acknowledgment's section. And you're right.

FOREWORD

by Charlotte Gerson

Andrew W. Saul is a man who enjoys his work. But do not be misled into thinking that the fun you will have reading this book makes its message any less serious. Dr. Saul is a committed activist and therapist who has brought sound nutritional information to thousands through his books, newsletters, and lectures.

Much has been written about nutrition and juicing, so Dr. Saul decided to write something different: "This is what I did." He has recorded a family saga that at times makes you laugh out loud and at times fills you with admiration for this charming medical teacher and his iron determination.

How much do we love our children? Enough to make them work hard hours, fighting off frogs and mice in an overgrown vegetable garden, and then drink the juices from their own organic produce? Enough to resist their complaints and overcome their (and our own) laziness? Enough to turn our backs on a totally unhealthy upbringing and start a relentless campaign to save them from antibiotics, vaccinations, pharmaceuticals, and chronic disease? That is how much Andrew Saul loved his children. The youngsters grew to college age without ever taking antibiotics and into maturity sharing their parents' values and valuing their sharing.

Much of the charm of Dr. Saul's story is in the humorous recollections provided by his daughter and co-author Helen Saul Case. Affectionately recalling her rebellious childhood, handled with creative blackmail and rewards by her wise and determined parents, she describes how "the system worked," since she continues the family tradition of juicing and teaching nutrition to her own children.

If all parents were able to benefit from the advice in this book, and were to make a habit of growing or purchasing a wide variety of organic vegetables to eat and juice daily, they could do much to avoid the terrible health problems that afflict children today.

Juicing is time invested in saving time. It is better to spend some happy hours in the garden and kitchen than to be miserable and sick in hospital or in a doctor's waiting room. Dr. Andrew Saul proves, by the rich and varied activities of his life, that if you are healthy you will have plenty of time for work and fun.

I might add that work *is* fun when you are helping people get and stay well.

INTRODUCTION

Why did we write this book, and why should you read it?

Here's why: modern medicine is primarily the study of what happens when you put pharmaceutical drugs into malnourished bodies. This book isn't going to change all of that, but certainly part of it. At the very least, when going into the ring to fight the champ, you do not want one hand tied behind your back. Pure and simple: this is why you need to drink your vegetable juice. You cannot afford not to. Do we have the sure cure for diseases? No. If we did, we'd be Surgeon Generals of the World, and it might have even been on Fox News.

Now the sermon is over. The rest of this book is going to be fun, and perhaps a bit weird. Both authors have taught junior high, and you can blame that surrealistic experience for some of the book's point of view. When you work with adolescent kids with attitude, it sort of rubs off.

The "juices" we will be speaking of are not recreational, sweet beverages. They are liquefied garden vegetables and other produce. They are good, substantial foods. And they are good for you. So, what's wrong with fruit juices? Nothing. It's just that vegetable juices are so much better: they contain far less sugar and are more nutrient-dense. They can prevent illness; they can heal illness; they can become a part of your family life. And believe it or not, the whole thing can be fun.

And we are going to show you why, how, and now.

———

CONFESSIONS OF THE DAD
WHO MADE HIS KIDS
DRINK VEGETABLE JUICES

First they ignore you,
then they laugh at you,
then they fight you,
then you win.
—MAHATMA GANDHI (1869–1948)

onfederate General Robert E. Lee never spoke of the Union Army
by name. He referred to his Yankee opponents as "those people."
When I (AWS) showed up with my little children at a family gathering,
we received the same epithet. "I don't know what to feed *you people!*"
my mother would say. "Mom, it's really okay," I would reply. "Just put
out what you want to serve, and we will choose what we want to eat."
Seemed simple enough to me, but our kids' vegetarianism seemed to
continually provoke response. It was bad enough that my wife and I
were veggies, but the children too? Somehow, that seemed beyond clan
comprehension. Even as a very young father, I knew that quoting
George Bernard Shaw doesn't work in situations like this: "Why should
you call me to account for eating decently?"[1]

Nor did authoritative quoting or anything like it work at holiday
gatherings. When we went with the out-laws, *er,* in-laws, to a summer
reunion, we invariably got odd looks from every picnic table within
visual range. All we did was eat everything except the grilled meats. At

Thanksgiving, we ate everything but the turkey. Easter was the works without the ham. But this was not seen as normal, and there was an undercurrent of *sotto voce* disapproval. Our fitness as parents was in question.

And this was *before* we started juicing. Then the pulp *really* hit the strainer, so to speak.

"YOUR KID IS ORANGE"

The worst thing that can happen if you drink a gallon or so of carrot juice a day—and I've done it—is that you'll turn orange. You will. This happened when my son was about two years old. He really liked orange, cooked winter squash like butternut squash and Hubbard squash. He liked squash a whole lot. He also liked sweet potatoes. How do you say "no" to that, and why would anyone want to? When you have a two-year-old who enthusiastically eats his vegetables, you kind of go with it.

My young son would eat a considerably larger amount of these foods than most adults. When you consider how little he was, he was indeed getting a proportionally massive quantity of squash and sweet potatoes. I even gave him canned pumpkin. My wife nearly went apoplectic, but the simple truth of it is that pumpkin is both healthy and tasty. Read the label and try a spoonful. It's the pie without the sugar and the crust. It is also ready to eat and safe, as it is heat sterilized (as all canned products are) and requires no preparation. And it was quicker and easier than thawing and cooking frozen squash, and that's not hard. (Well, the block of it is until you thaw and cook it.) Yes, opening a can of pumpkin and instantly being able to feed a hungry child has its advantages. Political correctness is not among them. Too bad. My son loved pumpkin every bit as much as squash, maybe more.

As a result, one day, my father-in-law said to me, "Your boy is orange."

I said, "No, he's not." I was used to it; he looked normal to me.

My father-in-law said, "No, he's orange. Look. Come over here and look at him under the light."

I did, and he was. I had an orange two-year-old. He was never sick.

You have to understand this: this was a healthy little kid, but he was orange. I thought, "I'm going back to the drawing board. I must have missed something somewhere."

So I got on the phone and called up a professor of biology I knew. I said to him, "I have an orange child here."

There was a pause, and then after a moment he said, "That's perfectly harmless. That's called *hypercarotenosis*. It's just an excess of the orange carotene, the pigment, in the skin." He was right. It's rather like sticking your finger in beet juice or spilling tomato juice on a white shirt. It's just coloring, a natural coloring. Indeed, carotene is actually used as a coloring agent in industry.

The professor continued: "All you have to do is not feed him any of the orange vegetables for a couple of weeks, and it will go away." Afterward, I read further into the matter to make sure I'd not done any harm. As a parent you certainly don't want to hurt your own kids. You do the best you can, and you're learning all the time. I was a young man with ample book learning but no experience. So I looked it up in the *Merck Manual*.

Just about every doctor has a *Merck Manual* in their office. It's sort of the Cliff's Notes of medical school. It's everything doctors learn in medical school condensed to about 3,000 pages. I looked up both hypercarotenosis and hypercarotenemia (high-carotene blood levels). The *Merck Manual* said—and still says, you can check online and see for yourself—that they are harmless. *USA Today* once described hypercarotenosis as an artificial suntan. I thought that was rather charming.

We backed off the squash and pumpkin, and in about two weeks, as the professor predicted, my son no longer looked like one. I had to say that because you have been waiting for it. The truth of it is, the orange coloring is very modest; it really does more resemble a suntan than the Great Pumpkin.

I now have a slightly orange granddaughter. She's healthy, too.

The last thing you want is a sick kid. The second-to-last thing you want is to discourage your child from chowing down on vegetables that are good for him or her. I do not recall any sickness during the Orange Child era.

So, to keep a good thing going, we started vegetable juicing.

Orange Kid: The Next Generation

Just like my (HSC) brother and I, with a diet abundant in pureed pump-kins, carrots (either cooked or juiced), soft sweet potatoes and prepared squash, my daughter couldn't escape being tinted orange at the tender age of one.

Folks thought she might be getting too much sun. And yes, my daughter did look "summery," but the sun was not to blame. Her summer attire con-sisted of light, long-sleeve clothes and floppy hats, we took advantage of nature's shade under massive trees, and, when necessary, sun block pro-tected her tender baby skin. She cer-tainly got some sun, but not enough to give her that fake-tan look that had

> The best way to get vitamin A, and the safest way, is through green leafy vegetables, orange vegetables, and their juices. Yes, green veggies con-tain a lot of orange carotene; it's just hidden behind a mass of green chlorophyll. You cannot overdose on vitamin A if you take it as carotene, because carotene is harmless.

people raising their eyebrows *at me*. With no discernible tan lines (I have changed enough diapers to know), I surmised that my baby girl was just a bit orange. She also was (and is) healthy.

Her pediatrician was shocked when she saw my daughter at her last wellness visit, and no, it wasn't because of her skin tone. Her doctor exclaimed, "Wow! She is only here for immunizations and well-visits!"

I smiled.

My baby girl smiled too, but she was probably just amused with the tongue depressor.

The Carrot Juice Moustache

Most parents have seen a "milk moustache" on their children's faces. Our (AWS) kids had bright orange "carrot moustaches." (If Mark Twain had juiced, just imagine.) That's how much carrot juice they drank, even as preschoolers. They also never had a single dose of any antibiotic. Not one, not ever. And they had pediatricians that they never met. Our family's physicians were in a group practice. Doctors came and went and we never met them. Just postcards announcing who was new, and who had retired.

And this went on all the way until the children went to college. There's not a lot of vegetable juicing going on in the dorms at your average institution of higher learning. That's all the more reason to start the kids right and early.

The carrot juice moustache: indeed, I have one now as I write this. Just finished juicing. Actually, you never really "finish" juicing. You kind of adopt it . . . and it you.

It was not always like that.

GROWING UP NOT JUICING

When I was a kid, supper came out of a can—or more correctly, from an assortment of cans. The dog's supper came from a can; the cat's food was canned as well. Everything came in cans; we had no freezer. It was the age of high-stacked pyramids of shiny cylindrical-steel supermarket specials, and my parents knew how to stock up. They bought by the case, storing cans of pretty near anything and everything in our "family room," a builder's euphemism for "upper basement of a split-level tract house." My father was no cabinetmaker, but by golly he could build shelves. It was these industrial-strength, scrap-wood shelves, packed to the rafters with A&P canned goods, that gave our family room its bomb-shelter survivalist motif. To my Berlin-Wall, Russia-has-the-H-bomb child's mind, there was an odd comfort in seeming to be prepared.

And we were. We were, after all, the only family in the neighborhood that bought tuna by the case, and we are not talking about a mere convenience six-pack: a case of chunk-light tuna was forty-eight cans. Then there was the canned creamed corn (not bad); canned lima beans (truly awful); canned mixed vegetables (damn near inedible); and my all-time nemesis, canned peeled white potatoes. These starch balls from hell were pasty, devoid of flavor, and just as likely devoid of nutrition. As far as I could see, most of these delicacies were purchased mainly because they were cheap. My mother and father scrimped and did not miss an opportunity for a "bargain," regardless of the consequences to the three of us kids. The grocery store manager abetted their pecuniary inclinations, providing a 10 percent case discount, and that was on top of the special sale pricing. My parents simply could not resist, and the packed, stacked shelves proved it.

There are people who would pay money at Vegas to play a game that was institutionalized at our house. It was "Unlabeled Can Dinnertime Roulette." One of the problems with canned goods is the quality of glue on house-brand labels. The labels inevitably came off during any kind of long-term storage. The problem, seemingly a trivial one, was compounded over the years as more and more cans were accidentally delabeled, consciously deselected, pushed to the back and forgotten. Periodically, in a spate of economy, my mother would send us downstairs to bring up "those" cans, and that would constitute the theoretical basis for dinner. My heavens, it was awful.

I really enjoyed eating at other kid's homes and did so at every opportunity. But those opportunities were entirely too few and far between. So we had to make do, and I am living proof that we did. I did not like the process. I was a finicky eater to begin with, and that was a luxury that was out of the question in our household. There were Children Starving in India, and Children in Africa Who Would Be Grateful for what was congealing on my dinner plate. Or so the legend and the house law went. Things we did not want to eat— things that *no* sentient being would want to eat—were called "eligible food" by my mother. The eligibility in question was for dessert, and this was no small incentive to down the indescribably indigestible. My mother might not have been an inspired cook, but she loved to bake. Pumpkin custard, egg custard, Boston crème cakes, pinwheel cookies, chocolate chip cookies, and homemade pies (Dad liked mince especially) were almost always on hand . . . one dinner at a time, of course. To miss dessert was like missing Halley's Comet or the Beatles on the *Ed Sullivan Show*. We steeled ourselves and ate without easily audible complaint.

Necessity Is the Mother of Juicing

My children will tell you that I am responsible for their juicing. Interestingly, they are responsible for my juicing. I never went near a juicer until I was in my twenties, had two kids, very little money, and absolutely no health insurance. I therefore had the strongest possible vested interest in keeping my children healthy. I literally could not afford to have a sick family. So, I bought a juicer at my friend's health food store to ensure the outcome we had to have.

Parents have an edge, and it is a good thing. The first rule of lion taming is that you have to be smarter than the lions. As a young parent I knew precious little, but I still knew more than my babies did. Generally speaking. Kids have instincts that also are real assets. One is the instinct to root, or suck for liquid. Breast milk, the original fresh mammalian juice drink, is sweet and infants absolutely love it. The sweet instinct carries through to fruits and ripe vegetables, which are also sweet. Juice them, and the result is even sweeter. (For those who think vegetable juices are *too* sweet, we will address glycemic content later in the book.) The sweet instinct is hardwired into us. Done right, it is using biology for our own good.

Candy Is Entirely Too Dandy

Aye, there's the rub: the search for sweet is easily perverted by candy and soda pop, as it was when I was a child. Stopping this is easier said than done; my parents tried to get me to eat right by offering meals that were pretty much devoid of junk food. Okay, Spam and cold cuts were no prizewinners, but my dad liked them, along with the occasional ginger ale as a holiday treat. His father loved ice cream, thank heaven, and grandpa insisted on generous portions when he visited. Even when grandparents were not there to rescue us, we had a lot of ice cream, at half a dollar for half a gallon, for the really cheap "Ann Page" stuff, A&P supermarket's house brand.

But it was never enough. That seek-the-sweet instinct is a strong one. As preadolescents, like junior Confederate raiders behind enemy lines, we also foraged. Behind our row of newly built houses was a low-lying stretch of Baltimore and Ohio Railroad tracks, three wide and miles long. This was bordered by a low-lying no-man's land of undeveloped brush, weeds, and cottonwood trees. The gully was our playground; our construction arena; our escape from parental presence. We built a tree fort (not to be confused with a mere tree house) and ate our summertime and weekend lunches up in the trees every chance we got. And, as bologna sandwiches somehow seldom satisfy, we foraged.

Up and down along the trackside were blackberry bushes in profusion. The thorns drove us to wear long sleeves even in July, but even the cuts were worth it. We found wild red raspberries bordering the nearby cemetery, unappreciated by our "quieter neighbors." Further down the tracks, one very much-alive neighbor had an unguarded cherry orchard, which we raided a few times until very nearly caught. Another neighbor had a bountiful plum tree that hung, heavy with fruit, conveniently over their fence line. Unlike the cherry orchard debacle, this made the produce kid-legal in our eyes. If we could reach it, we harvested it. And ate it. We were sometimes sufficiently energetic to gather enough berries to be able to sell the surplus . . . and take the profit straight to the candy store, of course. Once we cleared fifty cents. Even divided four ways, that bankrolled a nice sugar buzz for all. If it had just been a partnership, two of us could have been sick as dogs. Let me tell you how.

How to Get Sick for a Quarter

I was the neighborhood expert on overconsumption of cheap candy. As a little kid, if I had any money at all, I spent it on candy. At age six, I would walk a quarter mile each way literally to spend two pennies at the candy store. A nickel was substantial finance, and a quarter was the door to unspeakable decadence. We're talking over half a century ago, so you will have to adjust for inflation. But before you do, revel in how you could, and we routinely did, get sick for twenty-five cents.

Access to a tooth-shattering variety of penny candy was part of it, but that's for amateurs. Here's the *real* trick: two-for-a-penny candy. Red Hot Dollars, licorice, sour balls, and some other confections were two for a cent in 1961. So, you buy ten cents' worth. Good start: you now have twenty items in the bag and you still have fifteen cents in hand. Next, you buy two large Hershey bars at five cents each. Nestlé bars weighed one-eighth of an ounce less, so the decision was an obvious one. That's twenty cents spent, and your pancreas is already vibrating. But where this reaches the heights of genius is what you do with that final nickel. Surely, you want some pop, but Coke and Pepsi and Crush and Canada Dry and Nehi and Royal Crown and all the rest were ten cents a bottle. All except Dr. Pepper, which was seven cents. With two cents' deposit on the bottle, if you drank it there, it was only a nickel. Ta da!

Uphill Both Ways

Then there was school. We walked, every day. It was three quarters of a mile each way, and home for lunch. Four three-quarter-mile treks is three miles a day. That is on foot, all weather, crossing more than a half-dozen city streets, at age six, to get to first grade. You had to live over a mile from school to get a bus pass. Now you know where the sugar went.

School snack time was regulation. Graham crackers and milk are hard to criticize, except when the milk was warm and the crackers stale. During the interminable Rochester winters, enterprising teachers kept the milk cartons precariously balanced outside on the classroom windowsills. We had unsweetened, unflavored frozen "milk" shakes more than once. In fifth grade, our teacher experimented with our good judgment and said we could bring in our own morning snacks. The experiment would have been more successful without me in the classroom. I brought a fresh vegetable snack, which, to me, seemed perfectly portable, naturally nutritious, and a sure attention-getter: a whole raw onion. As I conspicuously consumed it, an uproar from my nearest classmates ended snack time for a month—for all of us. Kids can sometimes be pretty unkind, but the mere fact that I was not lynched at lunch proves that there is great compassion and tolerance in children.

As for that onion: why would the Twofer-a-Penny Candy Kid go for onions? Truth is, kids have other instincts than just for sweets. I actually liked raw vegetables enough to ask my mother to let me have my portion before she cooked them. She occasionally agreed. I still hate cooked celery. But the real question is, *why cook foods that can be eaten raw? And should be?* Somehow I knew that as a child. Maybe all kids have such innate understanding.

THE MALNOURISHED GENERATION

It was a time of rocket fins on cars, x-ray machines in shoe stores, and black-and-white classroom movies promising nuclear power and electricity too cheap to meter. But the 1950s also was a nutritional Dark Age. Propaganda for Victory Gardens and healthy soldiers ended when the Second World War ended. Pharmaceutical medicine was on the rise, and interest in vitamins, so keen since the 1920s, was out. The result? Babies of the 1950s, like me, were all vitamin deficient. Breastfeeding was then considered primitive, even unseemly. Bottle-feeding "formula" was the modern, scientific way.

But any man-made formula cannot possibly contain what men do not put in it. Truly, it is breast milk that is scientific. It is complete, and has been clinically tested for millions of years on billions of babies. Think of breast milk as juicing-food for babies, without having to buy the juicer or guess what to put through it. Babies like nursing. It's good for them, it's less expensive, it's easier for mom, and, like gravity, it always works. That word is *always*. And for backup on this point, I call your attention to the La Leche League, and the summary judgment of Professor of Pediatrics Robert S. Mendelsohn, M.D.: "The only women who cannot breastfeed are those who have had double radical mastectomies, or those who go to pediatricians." But back then it was not medically fashionable. I and my cooperative contemporary compatriot co-infants coast to coast were bottle-fed on formula that was inadequate and incomplete.

Typically, our mothers consumed too little folic acid while they were carrying us. Folate is abundant in raw food plants. *Folium* is Latin for "leaf." Folate is now well known to prevent birth defects such as spina bifida. I had slight spina bifida at birth, and like many other adults of my generation, it is still just noticeable if you know where to look. But back then, folic acid was not added to foods as it fortunately is today. Furthermore, 1950s formulas were not fortified with the B-vitamin biotin (sometimes known as B7). This too is a shame, as biotin was known since 1936 to be essential to the health of mammals. Guess what mammary glands provide? Biotin is only needed in small quantities, and the bacteria in your intestines can synthesize some. As for folate,

Popeye ate spinach so I did too. Even dogs and cats occasionally eat grass and greens. And it is not because they want to vomit. A modest amount of vegetable matter is good for them.

We were also vitamin E deficient, and so were our parents. In a way, it is amazing that we got here at all. *Health Culture* magazine for January 1936 said of vitamin E: "Its absence from the diet makes for irreparable sterility occasioned by a complete degeneration of the germinal cells of the male generative glands. [T]he expectant mother requires vitamin E to insure the carriage of her charge to a complete and natural term. If her diet is deficient in vitamin E . . . the woman is very apt to abort . . . It is more difficult to insure a liberal vitamin E supply in the daily average diet than to insure an adequate supply of any other known vitamin."[2]

Since the word *tocopherol* is taken from the Greek words for "to carry offspring" or "to bring forth childbirth," it is positively weird that, for decades on end, there was no government recommendation whatsoever for vitamin E for mothers and their babies and toddlers and teenagers. Yet as early as 1931, Philip Vogt-Moller of Denmark successfully treated habitual abortion in human females with wheat germ oil vitamin E. By 1939 he had treated several hundred women with a success rate of about 80 percent. A. L. Bacharach's 1940 statistical analysis of published clinical results "show quite definitely that vitamin E is of value in recurrent abortions."[3]

Yet when the Minimum Daily Requirements (MDRs) first came out in 1941, there was no mention of vitamin E. It was not until 1959 that vitamin E was recognized by the U.S. Food and Drug Administration (FDA) as "necessary" for human existence, and not until 1968 that any government recommendation for vitamin E would be issued. By then, I was thirteen. Yet, somehow my contemporaries and I must have unwittingly scraped together enough nutrients to survive. Vitamin E is found in very many foods but in very small quantities. A heaping cup of carrots contains, at most, about 1 international unit (IU) of vitamin E. Nuts and wheat germ are far better but, unfortunately, have a history of being relatively unpopular dinnertime entrees.

I honestly do not know how so many kids in the 1950s were conceived, carried, born, or grew once they hatched. Unfortunately, many still do not.

Even today, one in five pregnancies end in miscarriage. Perhaps repeated procreation, historically proven to be perennially popular, overcomes all odds. I'm here; so are my brothers. But although the Baby Boom boomed in the very teeth of lousy diet, better nutrition for mother and baby is still the right thing to do. And in our opinion, vegetable juicing is one of the easiest ways to obtain it. All roads may or may not lead to Rome, but in this book, every road, every story, every argument, leads back to that simple fact: vegetable juicing is really good for your whole family.

A Walk on the Nutritional Wild Side

Not everyone knows that bacteriologist Alexander Fleming, M.D., (1881–1955) wrote, "Penicillin sat on my shelf for twelve years while

---

"PUT YOUR HANDS UP AND WALK AWAY FROM THE VITAMIN E!"

"Any claim in the labeling of drugs or of foods offered for special dietary use, by reason of Vitamin E, that there is need for dietary supplementation with Vitamin E, will be considered false" (U.S. Post Office Department Docket No. 1/187, March 15, 1961).

On October 26, 1959, the U.S. government charged an organization known as the Cardiac Society with postal fraud for selling 30 IU vitamin E capsules through the mail. A four-day hearing in Washington, D.C., generated sufficient testimony to fill "four volumes totaling 856 pages. Seventy-six exhibits were received in evidence . . . for the consideration of the Hearing Examiner. His Initial Decision covers forty-two pages."

It is an oddity of history that, at the height of the Cuban Missile Crisis, the United States of America found both the reason and the resources to prosecute such a case as this. But it did, and the vitamin E seller lost. After this, all mail addressed to them was undelivered, and returned to the sender, with "Fraudulent" stamped on the envelope.

Today, you can now order vitamin E online or by mail. But this may change. Do an Internet search for *Codex Alimentarius* (Latin for "Book of Food") and learn how there is an international United Nations-sponsored effort to restrict nutritional supplements, restrict potency, restrict availability, and make them into prescription-only items.

I was called a quack. I can only think of the thousands who died need-lessly because my peers would not use my discovery." Juicing advocates and natural-health practitioners understand this all too well. Accept-ance of nutrient-based therapeutics has been decades long in coming. Health nuts, especially juicing nuts, have been criticized, even ridiculed, in their time. For many a year, as the bluesmen say, they paid their dues. As a young parent, I emulated the health nuts not because they were unappreciated, but because my personal parenting experience, year by year, proved them right. Not a single cell in the human body is made from a drug. All cells are made from nutrients. Fresh-vegetable, whole-some-food-based medicine makes good health and it makes good sense. Drugs do not.

If medical journals bloated with pharmaceutical advertising do not seem to get this, the public does. Everybody has seen a juicing info-mercial. Nutrition-based therapies make sense, good sense, common sense. Asked megavitamin physician and researcher Abram Hoffer (1917–2009), "If drugs make a well person sick, how can drugs make a sick person well?"

This question has been long been pondered. We even have mention in that classic medical text of the early 1960s: Ian Fleming's James Bond novel, *Thunderball*. British spymaster "M" actually lectures agent 007 that "All drugs are harmful to the system" and the denatured food we eat is little better since it "has had most of the vitamins boiled away, everything overcooked and denaturized." M concludes saying that "there is no way to health except the natural way." James Bond's unspo-ken response was to wonder, "What the hell had got into the old man?" Bond was clearly shaken, but not stirred. His diet remained unaltered.

"There is no way to health except the natural way." Sounds like something Grandma might have said. Indeed, "medical heretic" Dr. Robert Mendelsohn (1926–1988) maintained that one grandmother is worth two MDs. Two-time Nobel Prize winner Linus Pauling, Ph.D., (1901–1994) also had his own particularly direct recommendation. Dr. Pauling wrote that the following label caution should appear on every pharmaceutical product on the shelves: "Keep this medicine out of the reach of everybody. Use vitamin C instead!" To that, we would add, "And dust off your juicer and use it!"

PERHAPS THE MOST UNUSUAL GOURMET IN HISTORY

Not everyone uses a juicer. Michel Lotito, born in France in 1950, certainly did not. "Mister Eats Everything" began eating metal and glass when he was nine years old, by accident. Then he acquired the habit. According to the *Guinness Book of World Records,* his diet has included light bulbs, a supermarket cart (which took him four and a half days), entire TV sets, chandeliers, countless double-edged razor blades, many bicycles, and an all-metal, single-engine airplane. It took him an hour to eat an entire bicycle rim. It took him years to eat the airplane. But eat it he did.

Mr. Eats-Everything died at the age of fifty-seven. There is a lesson in here somewhere.

Carrot Team

Carrots contain a lot of carotene, and carotene is both healthy and harmless. There are several carotenes, the most famous of which is beta-carotene. Beta-carotene can be converted in your body into vitamin A whenever your body wants to. That is good. In many ways, carotene is a better source than the preformed oil (retinol) form of vitamin A. If you take the vitamin A as fish oil and you're possibly pregnant or thinking of becoming pregnant, that could be a problem. You don't want to take too much vitamin A as fish oil, especially the ladies who might be having a child, whether they know it or not. The way to sidestep the whole issue is to use the carotenes. It's the safe way to go for all ages.

Once in a while, a doctor will say, "No, you can't take carotenes because there was once a study in Finland that showed that carotene increased lung cancer." Let's settle this one. Dr. Abram Hoffer, a physician with an additional doctorate in biochemistry, called my attention to the fallacies in this study. I, therefore, found that the negative-carotene researchers studied people who were or had been heavy smokers. When we have a confounding factor like that, we can hardly blame the carrots. If you're wondering what causes cancer, is it carrots or Camels?

I'm pretty sure the cigarettes are the cancer risk and the carrots are not. Don't let anybody put you off carotene. Carotene is good for you. It's a very strong antioxidant. Grandma said to eat your vegetables. I'm saying to eat your vegetables, except I suggest you put them through a juicer. By the way, we have no financial connection with anyone who sells or manufactures juicers. (We also have no connection with anyone in the natural products or food supplement industries, and we have no connection with any vitamin company. We'd like to keep this book unbeholden and clear-cut.)

Everyone knows that carrots are good for you. We are emphasizing them at the outset because they are cheap, easy to juice, and taste really good juiced. But the rule is: you can juice *any* vegetable that you can eat raw.

PREGNANCY AND VITAMIN A

In *The Vitamin Cure for Women's Health Problems*, I (HSC) mention the importance of vitamin A: it helps fight off infection and it helps build your immune system. If pregnant, it is safest when ingested in the form of beta-carotene.

In addition to juicing, supplement your diet with vitamin A capsules, in the form of beta-carotene, especially on days when you don't juice. Vitamin A is an "immune enhancer,"[4] exactly the kind of thing needed to help strengthen your system. Getting your vitamins through juicing is ideal, but if you can't, taking a supplement works too.

If you are pregnant, the recommended dosages for vitamin A change, as large amounts of *fish oil* vitamin A can cause birth defects—but then again, so can vitamin A deficiency.[5] If you are pregnant, chat with your doctor before taking supplemental A, or just stick to carrot juicing. Beta-carotene (found in carrots, thus the similarity in name) is considered safe and nontoxic, even in large doses.[6] Beta-carotene converts into vitamin A in your body, and your body is smart enough to convert just the right amount it needs.[7]

FROM *TIME* MAGAZINE, DECEMBER 29, 1941

"Three new characters made of carrots (Dr. Carrot, Carroty George, Clara Carrot) have been photo-wired to London. They are advising the British that if they want to see better during blackouts, they had better munch carrots." These pro-carrot cartoon characters had been created, with wartime élan, by Walt Disney. (For more, and we mean a whole bunch more, information on the history of carrots, especially "Carrots in World War II," you will not want to miss the online World Carrot Museum at www.carrotmuseum.co.uk.)

JUICING: THE REAL STORY

You've seen those juicing infomercials on TV. They don't really do much for me, but the fact is that they're basically right. Fresh, raw vegetables are good for you.

Is this news? When you juice them, you have to understand what you're actually doing. When you juice vegetables, you're only doing two things: first of all, you're taking that vegetable and grinding it up so that, without cooking it, you're able to get all the nutrients out of the cells. Pick up a carrot sometime. If you were to get hit by a carrot, it would hurt. It's woody and hard. It has cellulose walls in there. These things are very strong.

It's the same with a parsnip, beet, or whatever. When you juice, you're breaking down all the cell walls and releasing all the nutrients, and you're doing that without cooking. Juicing gets you *better absorption*. You could eat five pounds of carrots, I suppose, if you took long enough. But you'd be doing nothing else. You could run five pounds of carrots through a juicer in about ten to fifteen minutes and get a quart and a half of juice. Then you could drink it, which is what I do. You get better absorption because it's been liquefied.

The second thing you get with juicing is you get *quantity*. I don't think I would eat five pounds of carrots, quite frankly. I just don't think I would do it. I think I'd get tired. My teeth would get tired. I'd get bored, and the taste buds would say, "Come on. Let's have something else."

When you juice, you can drink that quart and a half of juice down in no time. Juicing gives you more absorption, and you tend to take in a higher quantity. This means you get better results. Better absorption and higher quantity means better results, whether it's vitamin C or carrot juice. Don't let anybody dissuade you from juicing. Vegetable juicing is a tremendous help. In fact, the famous Gerson cancer therapy is based on juicing.

The Gerson Therapy

Dr. Max Gerson (1881–1959) was a German physician who had left Nazi Germany before it was too late to leave. By the way, all of his brothers and sisters died in the Holocaust. Gerson came over to the United States, fortunately for himself and for us, and began practicing in the Long Island area of New York. Dr. Gerson was known as a migraine doctor. He formerly had terrible migraines himself. He had tried all kinds of drugs and other therapies. Being a doctor, of course, he would have access to them. Nothing helped. Finally, Dr. Gerson decided to try nutrition.

Nutrition was the last thing he tried because, quite frankly, it's the last thing they teach in medical school. More correctly, they usually don't even bother to teach it in medical school. Most doctors have never had even one proper course in nutrition. Only a few have had two. I used to teach nutrition at a chiropractic college, and that chiropractic college required two courses. And I wouldn't say that two courses exactly make you a world-class expert. But necessity can. Dr. Gerson had to find something that would deal with his migraines and nutrition was the only thing he hadn't tried. By golly, when he started eating organic, fresh, unprocessed, natural, good foods from the garden, he found his headaches were relieved a great deal.

When he started putting these vegetables through a juicer and increasing absorption and quantity, he got rid of his migraines. People started coming to see Dr. Gerson to get rid of their migraines, and he became rather popular. Gerson noticed that his patients were not only getting over their migraines, but they were getting over other illnesses as well, including tuberculosis and several other very serious illnesses that he writes about in the books and publications mentioned in Chapter 4, where there is further discussion of the Gerson therapy.

There were people who came to Dr. Gerson and said, "Dr. Gerson, would you please treat my sister? She has cancer." Gerson said, "No, I will not. I am not going to get in trouble with the authorities. I'm not going to be known as one of those quacks who treats cancer. I'm sorry. I can't do that." They pleaded with him, and somehow they got to his heart.

Gerson realized that it was wrong not to do what you know might help. In fact, it's an axiom of medicine that you're supposed to do all that you can for the benefit of your patient. If a doctor does not do all they can, they're really not living up to their oath. Gerson decided to take the chance, and he started having cancer patients eat an unprocessed, organic, whole foods diet with no salt, virtually no sugar, reduced protein, and up to twelve glasses of assorted vegetable juices a day.

If a glass is 8 ounces, what is that, nearly 100 ounces? That's a lot of juice. It's a glass every hour. What he found was that the juices detoxified the body and helped the liver to recover. He believed the liver was the key organ to fight cancer in the body. Gerson was getting a very good cure rate. In fact, using juices and nutrients, Gerson's cure rate for terminal cancer was around 50 percent, which is extremely high. For malignant melanoma, his cure rate was spectacular. Dr. Gerson went before the U.S. Congress in 1946. They were talking about fighting cancer and what should be employed. Gerson said, "In addition to the other things, you want to consider nutrition." Gerson, unfortunately, was disregarded. Surgery, chemotherapy, and radiation were accepted and, more importantly, funded, whereas nutrition was put on the back burner.

Humanity has been suffering ever since, even though today every doctor knows that increasing vegetable consumption prevents cancer. But we are not acting accordingly. We have to change that right away. We have to get everybody juicing and eating right because this is what the body wants, and this is what brings you health. And it is best to start young.

Juicing Jumpstart

I am fascinated by animal behavior and always have been. Inherited instinct is a marvelous thing. I raised my children on property directly between two major migratory flyways near Lake Ontario in upstate New York. Watching the geese fly north over to Canada every spring, my children wondered if the geese were too early and might die from the cold. I, the biology teacher Dad, told my kids that the geese *had* to be right. Their lives depended on their instincts.

Human children may or may not have the instinct to seek out juiced vegetables. Personally, I think they do, but learn to fight it early. The trick is to steal a march on them and to get to them with behavior-modifying good examples first. Preferably, before they can say "no." As far as dissent goes, you give your kids what in British culture is called Hobson's choice: no choice at all. You give no choice here because you cannot take chances with your children's health. That is why you juice vegetables for them. The only better food is breast milk, and let's face it: babies grow out of that stage fast.

You know you are right because vegetables are good for you. So go ahead. If you do not comply with conventional medicine's doctrines, you had better make sure you can prove that you do not need them. Keeping kids healthy is the clearest possible win-win situation. Do not give your kids the chance to opt out of good health. You are bigger than they are, you are responsible for them, and you are smarter. Well, at least more experienced.

Making the less conventional health decision of loading up your kids on fresh vegetable juice—especially when they may not like it—means you are probably going to catch hell from somebody. If it's not from your kids, it will be from somebody else.

"Really?" you may ask. "Vegetable juicing isn't all *that* crazy. Kids often complain about eating veggies. Is juicing really going to raise eyebrows?" Sooner or later, yes. Insisting on certain health choices for your children isn't a walk through a tulip patch. As a parent you are imposing your right to give your child the nutrition you judge to be best. People may not always agree with you. I'm quite certain that they won't. You have to be strong and willing to stay the course through any opposition you might find. You are giving your kids vegetables. This is good. This is the way it should be. Put this in front of a jury of great-grandmothers and they will concur.

As frontiersman Davy Crockett said, "Be sure you are right, and then go ahead." Most of the country has it wrong when it comes to their diet. It somehow reminds me of my college psychology instructor who, speaking over a microphone to over 400 freshmen, would say, "If you cannot hear me, put your hand up."

Dick Gregory on Campus

Speaking of college, let me take you back to when I was a freshman. Comedian Dick Gregory came to our college campus to speak against the Vietnam war. The year was 1970, and the controversy was running high. Draft cards were burned and demonstrations shut down classes. I personally saw the student body president, from an overhead stairway, dump the contents of a fifty-pound sack of flour on two Marines at their recruiting table. My hair was a whole lot shorter than the student president's, but a good deal longer than the Marines'. At the time I was on the student activities lecture committee, and we knew full well we were bringing in a speaker who would be as inflammatory as he was funny. Anything else I knew of Mr. Gregory's politics came from reading *Dick Gregory: From the Back of the Bus* a few years earlier.

I was to be surprised. Gregory had pledged not to eat until the war was over. He started his fast at nearly 300 pounds and was down to 135. To save his life, his promise was amended to not eat any solids until the war was over. Viet Nam went on for years, so this was no wimp-out. He now lived on nothing but juice, fresh vegetable juice. In his lengthy speaking contract were written specifications about which and how many organically grown vegetables we were to provide for him. So our lecture committee had gone shopping for Mr. Gregory, and presented him with two large brown paper bags of fresh food. He carried them right into the student union's now very crowded press conference room, put the overflowing bags on the big dark-walnut table, and casually sat down.

I was four feet away from the man. The room was ablaze with the dazzlingly bright floodlights of TV reporters. Cameras whirred and clicked and the questions flew. As he quietly answered, Mr. Gregory calmly commenced juicing. I don't quite remember where the juicer came from, but there it was, all right. Cup after cup of orange or green drinks went into the man. The questions from the press stayed on his anti-war views. I don't recall any questions about his diet. It was weird to watch. I thought Mr. Gregory was off his rocker.

Years later, now pressed into responsibility as dad of two little children, I was rereading Mr. Gregory. Only this time, it wasn't his politics I was interested in; it was that darn juice thing. In *Dick Gregory's Natural Diet for Folks Who Eat: Cookin' with Mother Nature,* Gregory asserted that his kids had hardly ever been sick. I doubted that. Moreover, he wrote, they had never been vaccinated and they had never had any of the common and seemingly inevitable diseases of childhood. This I flatly disbelieved. But, driven by parenthood, I couldn't avoid being curious how he thought he'd managed that. I mean, sure he was wrong, but what if he was right?

In college, Professor John Mosher had taught me that scientists try all approaches until they find the one that works. At the time, I had listened quite dispassionately. But now I was faced with science made personal: I had a family. There not being any way to hurt kids with vegetables, I started juicing at home. Grumbling like refrigerators that are always running, my family nevertheless followed Mr. Gregory's health footsteps. (My daughter's grumbling follows later in this book.)

In total, it was successful. My kids got all the way into college and never had a single dose of any antibiotic. I have said that before. I say it a lot, because it is important.

WELL, IT'S CERTAINLY NOT GENETIC

We cannot teach people anything; we can only help them to discover it within themselves.
—GALILEO GALILEI (1564–1642)

When I (AWS) taught at New York Chiropractic College, I was known as "The Juicer." I gave a huge number of quizzes to my clinical nutrition students, and was probably known by some other names as well. But how did it all start? Who is this masked man with the carrot juice moustache? Here's the background story that resulted in, among other things, this book . . . and, in generational succession, its authors.

JUICER'S MOTHER

Although she was only thirty-six when I was born, my mother, Jean Chamberlin Saul, thought that a bit old. Perhaps it is a generational thing; today, many couples wait to have kids. I recall more than one occasion, when she was feeling weary, she told me the reason was that I was the "child of grandparents." She had good reasons to be weary. One was that she had epilepsy. It was managed with medication, which made her tired. Plus, I was not the firstborn; I had two older brothers. Not only that, she might have had enough to do if she'd had just me to care for. I was ten pounds, nine ounces at birth. That's a big baby. Throughout my infancy, whenever she took the bus down-town, which was frequently, she carried me on her hip like a Colt .45 Peacemaker.

I was not a hyperactive or high-maintenance child by any means, but I certainly was a motormouth. My father maintained that I started talk-ing early and never shut up. I recall him describing me as having been vaccinated with a phonograph needle. My mom is at least partly to blame. She had graduated from college before World War II and taught high school. She taught me to talk, and with competition from two older siblings, I learned to speak up or lose out.

My mother set good examples for me early in life. Even before I was of school age, I recall that when my mother took off her kitchen apron and started pushing the dinette chairs out of the way, it was time for the *Jack LaLanne Show*. Of course she had to turn on our ancient TV a good five minutes ahead of time, to let it warm up. I usually stuck around for the program, mostly as an excuse to see Lalanne's big white German Shepherd dog, Happy. But my line of work today shows just what a strong, if subliminal, impression the incredibly cheerful, incred-ibly agile Dr. LaLanne had made on me. That is not a misprint: he was a chiropractor. Jack Lalanne was the first TV exercise guru, and one of the first to subsequently come out big-time in favor of raw food juicing.

Mom was an avid swimmer both for fun and for exercise. In her sixties she could, and did, swim a mile nearly every day. My father could not swim a stroke. Still, he took her to the "Y" and sketched while he waited for her poolside. He was basically there to make sure the lifeguards were on the ball.

She set other very positive examples as well. City buses were crowded in those days. We were nearing our stop one evening, and working our way through the standing-room-only aisle to the door. Squatting down close to the floor was a boy about my age. Actually, he was sitting on a shoeshine kit, an obviously homemade wooden box with the expected contents. But he was black, and that stood out in busses going to our all-white neighborhood. He was also not much older than I was, and I was seven. The bus was really packed, and it took us a moment to pass him. As we did, I saw my mother slip him a dollar bill. Absolutely no one saw her do it, and she never said a word. I heard him very quietly say, "Thank you." As we walked home from the bus stop, I asked her why she had given him so much money for a ten-cent shine that she did not even get. To a kid, a buck was a lot back then, and by golly she never gave me one. She answered, "That boy is not shining shoes for himself. He is helping his family." To this day, when I see a dollar bill, I think of my mother.

In case this seems tenuously patronizing, I'd like to mention that my mother put serious money where her ethics were. I saw what she put in the collection plate at church, although she had it tightly folded up so you had to watch carefully. That is not especially remarkable, but I think this next act truly was. When our house went up for sale, among the people who came to look at it was a young African American couple. My mother was very impressed with them and told my father, and then the real estate broker, that she wanted to sell the house to the black couple. My father was fine with it, but the agent was not. He literally said, smiling all the while, "You simply cannot sell to them." My mother asked why, and the reason was color and nothing but. My mother said if she could not sell the house to them, she would not sell at all. She immediately took the house off the market, and we stayed put. Across half a century, I remember this.

The first copy of Betty Freidan's *The Feminine Mystique* that I ever saw was on my mom's bookshelf. I was about eleven or so. With a title like that, I figured it was a dirty book. I thought about reading it. After all, she did have a copy of *Lady Chatterley's Lover,* which I *did* read at an inappropriately early age. Not to worry: it was the 1960s American-expurgated version, so heavily censored that it was utterly inoffensive to anyone. Boring, too. I later learned to appreciate both books, for rather different reasons.

When she was a teenager, the girl who would much later become my mother firmly believed she would be the first woman president. She went to college in the 1930s, and few women did so. Her politics were and remained blatantly liberal: she was vociferously opposed to the Vietnam War. She wrote to the President every single day telling him to end the war now. This is not the slightest exaggeration: she wrote *every* day, consuming stacks of stamped postcards in the process. (Postcards were a penny cheaper to mail than an envelope.) She bought postcards in bulk, and when I said "every day" that included Sundays, so *two* postcards went out on their way to the White House on Mondays. With three boys, and having herself lived through World War II with my dad in the Army, my mother was not about to let up on this. It's a good thing Mom was a Democrat, or President Johnson would have *really* been in for it. As it is, I suspect she to be the reason he did not stand for re-election in '68.

Home Cooking—Oh, No

An inspired activist, yes; however, my mother was not an inspired cook. We ate a lot of meatloaf and a lot of frankfurters. We chowed down on white bread, which supposedly, somehow built strong bodies twelve ways. For dinner, Mom opened packages and cans . . . and then cooked them even further than the packers and canners did. Boy, did my mother cook, and overcook. Everything. Once I asked her why. "That's the way your father likes it," she said. Many years later, I finally marshaled the nerve to ask my father why he liked everything overdone. "Because that's the way your mother makes it," he answered. D'oh! I'd been living in an O. Henry story.

On the other hand, my mother was at least partly orthomolecular. Having opened the cans, she drank the juice the vegetables were packed in, or put it into homemade soups. My brothers and I each had to take a multivitamin every day, long before it was popular. "Take it now," she'd say, "before it rolls away." We never had a day without some sort of fruit juice, nor a day without whole grain cereals at breakfast.

The orange juice was okay, but I was not wild about grapefruit juice and prune juice, my mother's passion, freaked me out totally. When we had grape juice, it was watered down 50/50 because it was so expensive, and incidentally because it was so sweet. I accepted Wheatena, Ralston, or oatmeal as long as I could, and did, put sugar on it. Pancakes were great, and I loved waffles. Both were, to me, essentially maple-syrup delivery devices. My mom's ancient waffle iron, presumably passed down from Thomas Edison himself, was as large as a toilet seat, hot enough to broil a large mammal, and took enough amperage to make a prison warden wonder who had just walked their last mile. So, on those rare mornings when we had waffles, they were usually overcooked. When I was a kid, eating was a necessary evil. "Well done," at least in my experience, is the ultimate oxymoron. My mother could have burned ice cream if it were possible. A former history teacher, she simply lacked passion for cooking. Her casual disregard of any advances ever made in culinary science is approaching the legendary.

And she was relentlessly, creatively frugal. All food containers, bottles or cans, were rinsed to get the very last speck of nourishment out of them, and the rinse water added to dinner somewhere, usually in the soup or snuck into the ketchup. I did not know ketchup was supposed to be thick until I dined out. When a roll of film was used up, she would carefully wind the film to get an extra exposure. No kidding; this worked, at least with the old 616 black-and-white film. Eastman Kodak repeatedly sent us seven pictures from a roll that took six. She once had space for only one more photo, wanted to get the roll developed right away . . . and took a picture of the inside of our refrigerator. If there is a Nobel Prize for Surrealism, I have a nomination.

Years ago, as a preteen, my daughter profiled her for a school assignment, saying:

"In my house, the story has often been told of the gray Jell-O. When the flavors cherry and lime were mixed, a wonderful flavor resulted. But it was a horrible sight. Of course my Grandma Saul didn't mean for that Jell-O to be gray, but with only one box of each color, the double batch of Jell-O did not come out just right."

I would like to point out that hoof-derived desserts were a part of my childhood, but not that of my kids. "Gray" really makes you stay away.

Mom also mixed partly open boxes of breakfast cereal "to save space." I was raised on Cheerios, cornflakes, Wheaties, puffed rice, shredded wheat, and Grape Nuts . . . all in the same bowl. And on top of this, and again to save money, our family drank regular whole milk that was mixed with dry skim milk, 50/50. When we complained about the weak, watery consistency, my mother added more powdered skim milk to the point that it would not dissolve. Comedian Bill Cosby was famous for saying that he could not get down a lump of hot cereal. For me, I have a permanent aversion to lumpy beverages.

Like many kids of the '50s, we were compelled to eat liver. No muscle tissue, or internal organ a turkey ever had, was wasted. It all went into soup. Such time-honored cooking behaviors result in a reduced loss of vitamins and minerals. Today, I recognize "soup" as a dilute, precooked meat-and-vegetable extract. Back then, I simply thought she was a little nuts.

The moment Dad walked into the house after work, she met him at the door and he had a glass of orange juice stuck into his hand along with a Kodak vitamin pill (employee price: one dollar for 100 capsules) plunked in his mouth before he could say, "What's for dinner?" And since "What's for dinner?" was such a fruitless question anyway, everything (including liver) being uniformly overcooked into tastelessness, the pill no doubt did him much good. Same for us: we rarely went to the doctor; at five dollars a visit, it was "too damned expensive." When we did go, it usually had to be for a condition serious enough to require a tetanus shot or something even my father could not bandage.

JUICER'S FATHER

There was not a lot my father *couldn't* bandage. He practically rebuilt our combat-worn tomcat, Tony, on a regular basis. Tony got his name from being striped, so we named him after the famously extroverted cereal box tiger. He was the terror of neighborhood dogs as well as neighborhood cats. He would depart on fighting and mating binges that would span the better part of a week, and then show up home again. He was invariably in bad shape. Torn ears, open wounds, exposed muscle. During his feline benders, Tony clearly got the you-know-what kicked out of him, but I am reasonably sure we would not have wanted to see the other cat—or dog, squirrel, woodchuck, or armored-fighting vehicle.

My father's remedy of choice was hydrogen peroxide solution. Pa went through this by the quart. He took a contrite Tony down to the basement laundry tub and doused the cat with it. Once, the cat got skunked. Pa took the cat downstairs and this time immersed it in tomato juice. (See? This is still a book about vegetable juicing.) In case you think it's a myth, let me assure you that it really works. However, there is nothing on earth more pitiful than a wet, tomato-juiced cat.

Dad would have made a good paramedic and, once, he really had to be one. My hometown of Rochester, New York, is widely known for its wretched snowy winters. At times, Pa took the bus to work, and had a short walk from the bus stop to our house. Halfway home from the bus stop, there was a city sidewalk plow, really a tractor with an over-sized snowblower in front, that had been clearing the walk of at least two feet of new snow. The operator was trying to clear a stick or ice chunk from the blades with his heavily booted foot. The only problem was that the fellow had left the machinery running, and it was stronger than he thought. It took the end of his foot clean off, boot and all. There was blood gushing everywhere, scarlet spatters all over the white snow. Pa never missed a step. Instantly, he grabbed the man, pushed a big handful of snow onto the wound, and held it there. He carried the fellow to the nearest house, a two-family orange brick apartment. He pounded on the door, an old man opened it, and in they went, blood and all, all over the man's carpet. An ambulance was called. The man lived. I never found out what happened to the man's toes.

An Artist's Life

Dad was great in a crisis, but he was often impatient. Some people read while they wait for something. My father sketched. Constantly. For over twenty years, he kept a daily self-illustrated diary he called "Sketch-notes." It ran to some fifty-five volumes, including many thousands of quick sketches, comments, and watercolors on all conceivable topics. His notebooks at times are reminiscent of an almost Leonardo DaVinci-like rambling but entirely serious visual inquiry into the world around us. Sometimes, the drawings are just stream-of-consciousness cartoons done while my dad sat at the kitchen table, at a meeting, or in a waiting room. He sketched from his car in a parking lot, or at a stoplight or drive-up window. I like these the best. They are his take on his own life, seen through his own eyes.

My father also produced a considerable number of more formal watercolor, acrylic, or oil paintings. I think his best work may have been his quick watercolor sketches. These never took him longer than about twenty minutes, usually much less. Most of his watercolors are copies of, renditions of, or tributes to the work of his favorite masters. Chief among these would be the French and American Impressionists. He was especially keen on the circa 1900 American "Ashcan School" of artists who liked to draw just about anything, and did.

Just like Pa did. He would sketch what he saw, sketch what he thought, and sketch what he read. His work constitutes a slice of American life, from the start of the Second World War until a few weeks before his death in 1996.

A Boy of Summer

Like so many other boys, my father wanted to be a big-league baseball pitcher, and he came halfway close to making it. When still a teenager, he played semipro and pitched for a sub-bush league team in New Jersey. He tried out for the Yankees, but his fastball wasn't fast enough for the majors. But he did all right in the minors. Dad's greatest boys-of-summer moment was probably when he struck out Bobby Brown, twice in one game. Bobby Brown went on to become a World Series Yankee, a physician, and the president of the American League. Dad went on to become an artist.

While baseball's loss may ultimately have been our gain, my father had a pretty humble beginning to his art career: he was a sign painter during the Depression years of the late 1930s. He once had a job lettering a set of display windows for a local merchant. After he'd been outside on the job for a while, there was some kind of disagreement about payment, and the store owner said he would not pay. My father finished the job anyway. Now you are going to think this is a holier-than-thou story, but it is not. My father intentionally had used water-soluble paint, and the first time it rained, the lettering washed off in a blurry slurry of color.

After enlisting for service in World War II, he rose to the rank of sergeant. Twice. The first time he was promoted, he was AWOL, on the train to New Jersey to see his first-born child without a pass. When he got back, they canceled his promotion. He quickly made sergeant again. After honorable discharge, he became a draftsman. With variations on this theme, he would continue so until his retirement in 1986. He called this "tight" work, and though he was a fine illustrator, he did not especially enjoy industrial drawing. He preferred to paint, fast and loose, often dispensing with a brush altogether and using only a palette knife. Or, he would make a quick line drawing somewhere, probably on his lunch hour, and later add watercolor to it at home. His Spartan ground-floor studio at our home was also known as "The Kennel," because the family dog slept there at night. You have not lived until you've experienced the combined scents of turpentine and wet dog.

Life with Father

When I was little, my dad used barn paint on our house because it was a buck cheaper per gallon and, he believed, longer lasting than regular house paints. We had the only barn-red house in the neighborhood, and maybe even the city. Pop also made a large wood and metal star to display on our white front door at Christmas time. He painted it with the red barn paint, too. Imagine, if you will, the overall patriotic effect of a bright-red house, with a bright red star on the door . . . during the post-McCarthy era. Dad (who was fortunately well-known as a solidly American World War II veteran) finally realized the humor of the whole thing, and painted a one-inch green border around the star.

In addition to when he was sixteen feet up on an extension ladder, I watched him paint a lot. It was not because I was a dedicated, precocious observer. It was due to the fact that Pa painted practically all the time. He sketched while in church. He drew after (and during) meals. He painted signs and posters for charities and civic organizations, always free of charge. He lettered trucks for friends and neighbors. He also taught mechanical drawing for a time, briefly at the college level and even more briefly in high school. As a father with a wife and three sons, he went back to school and earned a master's in art history.

Middle-Aged College Man

When my father was a forty-one-year-old undergrad at the University of Rochester, I went with him on a geology class field trip to Jaycox

Run in Geneseo, New York, to dig fossils. I was seven. What a crushing bore that was, until one of his classmates dug up a trilobite. Whoo hoo. I also went to his graduation. The commencement speaker was the down-and-not-even-governor-of-California Richard Nixon.

Pa worked hard at the U of R, where he felt somewhat outclassed. He often was. I remember how hard he worked. He illustrated his own classroom notes so he could understand things visually. For his term papers, he worked even harder. His handwriting was exemplary, and yet he typically paid a typist to ensure a proper final version. At the "brain factory," as he liked to call "The University," Warren Saul earned a lot of C-plusses and B-minuses. His exam books, all of which he kept, show that he was no scholar. But he became one.

After earning, and I do mean earning, his bachelor of arts in geography, he went on to complete a masters in art history. My mother never wavered from maintaining her view that he did that to one-up her. Mom had been a teacher, you remember, and had a BA in History from Montclair State in New Jersey. She taught us the Montclair State football fight song when we were toddlers. If Montclair is ever playing any other team on the planet, I will root for the other team. Nothing personal, of course.

For one shining moment, my father rose spectacularly above academic mediocrity. He was writing a paper on Rembrandt's "Anatomy Lesson of Dr. Tulp." He would later cartoonize this famous painting at my request, and make it into the comical cover illustration for my second book, *Paperback Clinic*. It was a joke that almost no one ever got . . . except Pa and me. But anyway, Pa had a flair for the thorough, if not for the dramatic. He decided to check and see if Rembrandt got it right. So, Pa arranged to attend a human cadaver dissection at U of R's medical school. He gowned up and watched closely. Rembrandt was right: there are two sets of arm tendons, and the anatomy is accurate. However, he wrote, Rembrandt was not accurate in his portrayal of the appearance of the dead body. The color and, well, "lifelikeness" of the cadaver are artistic license. My dad was first to verify the one, and comment on the other. He aced his paper.

Then he had nightmares for months.

Maturity and Some Immaturity

For a consummate artist who could discern two dozen different shades of blue, Pa had incredibly bad taste in wardrobe. Oh, he could put on a dark suit and do the Kodak thing okay; it's what he wore when he was not at work that was enough to give Calvin Klein a coronary. He would wear plaids with checks, bright red pants with bright blue jackets, and brazenly loud bow ties with anything. The most outrageous outfit he ever wore, in my opinion, was his pajamas. My mother liked to sew. She was not particularly good at sewing, but made up for it with sheer inventiveness. Inventions are not always successful, my father the patent draftsman would tell you, but that does not stop inventors. Neither did such constraints as good taste stop my parents. When my mother made my dad terry cloth pajamas, she must have been low on material. The pajamas turned out Bermuda-shorts length, with wild, patterned green pockets cut from an entirely different fabric. Perhaps those pockets were not quite big enough to hold volume one of *Encyclopedia Britannica,* but it would have been a near thing. The worst part of it was that Pa absolutely loved them, and to prove it, wore the pajama pants in public. No, that was not quite the worst part; this was: he took me with him. When I was in ninth grade. To the neighborhood public library. Where my friends were.

I knew what was coming but was powerless to prevent it. The man whose best-known family phrase was, "Don't talk while I'm interrupting" was not to be dissuaded by the likes of me. Off we went to the Charlotte Branch of the Rochester Public Library, me hunching way, way down into the foam front seat of our sea-green 1960 Chevy.

When we got to the library parking lot, I deliberately dragged behind, as far as humanly possible. It was looking good: I was thirty feet back now as we approached the front double doors. Up the steps he strode; back on the sidewalk I slowly slunk. He opened the door, and in full view of the world, called back to me in his never-soft voice, "C'mon, Andrew!"

Oh, good grief. I followed him in and yes, right at the first lobby table were several of my friends. My memory blanks after that. I understand that is what post-traumatic stress can do.

When I was a boy I was infamous for waking up as early as 2:30 on Christmas morning, and almost never later than 4 o'clock. As my dad would be up past midnight decorating, he was for some reason not fully appreciative of my enthusiasm. As the decades passed and I had a family of my own, Pa started waking up earlier and earlier on Christmas morning, just as I had in my youth. It got so that he and my mother would open their presents Christmas Eve. They simply could not wait. There is something rather charming about that.

Pa loved the music and clowning of Spike Jones. He did a remarkably good impression of actor Peter Lorre in the song "My Old Flame." A natural born master of ceremonies, Pa could tell a good joke, or a bad one, and get good audience response. Once in a while he took center stage at home, although it was crowded under that spotlight with my brothers and me. The best mealtimes were when he told stories about being in the Army.

The Measure of a Man

Most of my father's professional life was spent behind a drawing board at Eastman Kodak Company. He executed many, many patent drawings during this time. Although patent illustrators are not allowed to sign their work, Pa did so anyway. He used Morse code, and concealed a "W. E. Saul" into each drawing's broken shading lines. So, if you really want to, you can go to the Patent and Trademark Library in Washington and find just which ones he did.

Before and especially after his retirement in the mid-1980s, Dad did many art lectures, free of charge, for churches and clubs. He usually talked about the architecture of the building the group was gathered in. Pa could tell you the construction date of any private or public building to within five years either way. He was never wrong.

Over time, these lectures turned into live how-to demonstrations. Pa insisted that to know how to paint, you first have to know how to draw. All the while explaining what he was doing and why, Pa would paint a picture in less than half an hour. His favorite subject? The *Titanic* leaving on its maiden voyage from Southampton. He was very interested in ocean liners. This is likely not only because he was a boy during their heyday, but also because the burning wreck of the liner *Morrow Castle* was beached within an easy walk of his New Jersey home when he was only thirteen.

I always knew my dad was a great artist, but I did not know why until I took art history at Brockport State. One day the instructor was showing the quick sketches of Rembrandt. I stared up at the lecture hall screen, and then I saw it. By golly! My dad had the same economy of line, the same lightning drawing speed as did the great master. I told Pa this, and he of course dismissed it. But after that, when we visited, he brought me photocopies of all his new sketches. And what's more, the man who so liked to quip, "If I want your opinion, I'll give it to you" actually did ask for my opinion on them. That is a moment we had for the ages.

For years, I remember Pa saying that when he retired, he was going to play golf every morning, and do paintings every afternoon. His surviving sketchbooks confirm that he kept at least the second part of that pledge to the letter. In later years, his hands and fingers were a never-ending sore spot for him, and after nine operations, he sold his golf clubs. However, he never got rid of his pencils, brushes, or pens. He kept right on drawing.

Of his thousands of surviving paintings and sketches, the online free-access archive at www.doctoryourself.com consists mostly of my favorites that were small enough to scan into a webpage. For every item there, a hundred more are waiting to be seen.

I do go off on tangents, by nature and also because my students and readers seem to respond positively. It is time for this digression from juicing to come home. After he retired, my dad finally started juicing. In my book *Doctor Yourself,* I have described how my mom got rid of her arthritis by eating fresh raw sprouts daily. But these events were to be many years in the future.

Well, that's my story and I am sticking to it. This is what it was like to be raised in a family where vegetable juice—and nearly everything else—came out of a can. And now, in the interest of equal time, the next chapter contains some choice words from my daughter.

3

CARROT JUICE KIDS

If you have a garden and a library,
you have everything you need.
—MARCUS TULLIUS CICERO (106 BC–43 BC)

Today is February 28, 2011, and my (HSC) nine-month-old daughter just had her first taste of carrot juice—and she liked it. She's far too young to be judgmental, but let's just give it some time.

When I was growing up, I'm pretty sure none of my friends were drinking their vegetables. Even if they claimed to drink V8 (probably mixed with a dab of chocolate ice cream, a squirt of ketchup . . . oh, and a greasy French fry on a school lunch tray while classmates placed bets—assuming of course someone's parents were actually silly enough to put V8 in their son or daughter's bagged lunch thinking they would actually drink it for anything less than a dollar), I would argue that V8 is about the same as drinking salty pasta sauce, and nothing like what my brother and I were getting at our house. If my parents had handed me something to drink that came prepackaged, fully endorsed and branded, I wouldn't have considered myself as ill-used. The unadulterated vegetable slurry they were tossing together in our little kitchen wasn't even close to V8. It was way different. And it was weird.

I was convinced that having to knock down a glass of homemade carrot juice was some sort of cruel and unusual punishment. Vegetables belong in a salad, not liquefied in a glass. Fruit juice made sense. Carrot juice did not. It was just so *strange*. And the fact that we drank it made *us* strange, and I assure you being labeled as such is a risky proposition in grade school. So, we told no one. I mean, if it was "normal," why couldn't you buy it at the store like that can of V8?

Well, you could—sort of. In the "old days" the only way you'd find carrot juice on your grocer's shelves was in a can. (I doubt anyone was cracking open a frosty container and taking a refreshing sip.) The stuff would be weeks, if not months old. It was about as tasty as you might imagine old vegetable juice in a tin might be—pretty bad. I'm sure nobody was buying it. And to their credit, my parents didn't either, but this didn't make us kids feel any better.

Times have changed, and now you can actually buy refrigerated, bottled carrot juice that is sweet and yummy. You have to pay for the privilege, but the prepackaged version isn't that much more money than homemade, and the dirty work has already been done. Those of you who regularly purchase whole carrots (it pays to buy fresh, organic carrots to get the best flavor) may notice that sometimes they are very sweet and yummy, and other times they can be downright bitter and bland. Since whole carrots can be inconsistent in their yumminess, bottled carrot juice (CJ) can be even tastier than what you can make. It's not raw, and therefore lacks the benefits of the freshly prepared concoction streaming from your juicer, but it'll do nicely in a pinch. When it's less than convenient to haul our heavy juicer around with us, my husband and I will buy carrot juice from the store. This is handy during the holidays when we are most assured to be stuffed with all sorts of treats when visiting relatives, but not so many vegetables. We make sure to stock our motel fridges with a few emergency quarts. Even if you didn't like the idea of ingesting orange liquid, it would be really hard to turn down this new store-variety of carrot juice for any other reason than prejudice; it's really good. Really. Disbelievers may want to give it a try.

Not everyone has an open mind of course. One summer afternoon I was chugging down a refreshing bottle of ready-made CJ, and my father-in-law, in response to the bright carroty liquid, wrinkled his nose and pronounced, "Ew! What are you drinking!?" I wasn't about to let him get away with disparaging my food choice, especially a healthy one like this. Certainly, he meant no harm, but I wasn't about to take a comment like that and do nothing about it. He'd probably be one of the first people in line who would say he need not be "over-managed." Since I don't know any better, I often suggest to him helpful little tidbits of information, and he politely smiles, and proceeds to do whatever he wants, as it should be I suppose. However, it seemed only fair that his critical commentary get an appropriate response. So I poured a glass and demanded that he drink it.

No amount of my talking was going to change my father-in-law's mind about carrot juice, but to his credit, cornered and chagrined, he sipped a quarter cup's worth and admitted that yes, it was actually very good. For a fella that's never had a drop of carrot juice in the sixty-five years he's been on this planet, it shows even skeptical folks can come around.

I was so embarrassed to be drinking carrot juice when I was growing up. As far as I'm concerned, I was lucky to get through my teen years without being tarred and feathered. And here I am now, drinking that same loathsome, torturous beverage. Except now it's just normal, and I happen to like it and what it does for me. I drink a glass several times a week. So does my husband. And so does our daughter, in a sippy-cup of course.

Someday our daughter will complain about the things we feed her. Goodness knows she'll have to have *something* to fret about when she is young. It may as well be her spectacular diet.

IT'S A MATTER OF MOTIVATION

My parents rarely bought ready-made desserts. Sweets were not stocked in our house, unless you count Dad's secret stash of the after-Christmas sale of Russell Stover Assorted Creams. Okay, we had the occasional need to buy that bag of day-old doughnuts or a cheese Danish or two, but in general, our family's access to prepackaged goodies was very limited. The problem was a simple one: if we had it in the house, we were likely to eat it. So the first rule of good health was simply to keep the junk food out of reach. What is the first thing we go for when we are hungry? The quick-fix sugar boost is hard to resist. It takes time, motivation, and patience to prepare a good-for-you meal instead; it takes an immense amount of willpower to choose the healthy snack over finger-lickin' tasty treats, let alone drag out a juicer and proceed to liquefy the contents of your refrigerator's veggie drawer. And then drink it.

If my parents were going to make us knock back all these juiced vegetables, and then allow us to have "what we wanted within reason" afterward, in my mind there had to be a treat worth eating to make this all worthwhile. There had to be something super tasty we could possibly get our hands on if we were good kids and drank the juice like we were told. (If your child drinks several pounds of juiced carrots, are you really going to deny them a cookie? Of course not.) Therein lay the brilliance behind the plan. We may not have had any candy in the house, but we did own granulated sugar . . . and powdered, unsweetened cocoa. There were flour, eggs, and milk. If I wanted to have goodies in the house, I was just going to go ahead and make them—from scratch. I knew my mom and dad were suckers for desserts (aren't we all?) and homemade ones take the cake, so to speak. Homemade baked goods were free of chemicals, preservatives, food paint, and other additives: strong selling points for health-nut parents.

I didn't really want to bake all the time. But I wanted even less to be without the motivation needed to chug glassfuls of vegetables.

My folks were becoming expert juicers. So I became an expert baker. Okay, perhaps "expert" is a bit presumptuous, but for a twelve-year-old, I made one darn fine dessert. My chocolate chip cookies came out moist and chewy; brownies were soft and cakey; pies came out toasty and flaky. Making "perfect" desserts was out of sheer necessity, mind you. If I ruined my confections in the oven, and wasted all those materials, I would not have been given the opportunity to make more. Everything had to be as perfect as possible.

And it worked.

It will with your kids too! If your kids drink veggie juices without complaint, that's fantastic. As for the rest of them, it doesn't hurt to dangle a carrot out there, I mean cookie, to get them to put down an abundance of nutritious food.

But Don't Forget, or Else . . .

Once a week my parents would schedule a date night. Sometimes this would involve preparations such as hiring a babysitter, setting aside for us some healthy snacks in the fridge like carrot sticks and deviled eggs, and making it clear that our 7 o'clock bedtime was still in effect. Then they'd head out to dinner and a movie. However, more often than not, it was just a whole lot easier for them to put us kids to bed, or set us to some other task, order a pizza, and watch a cheap rental film on the couch instead.

Mom and Dad felt it was important to have time together and something special just for the two of them; it's not like we didn't get pizza as a family. But, the frequency at which pizza actually showed up on our dining room table was nowhere near the number of times my older brother and I could have eaten it. Date night or not, he and I wanted in on that pie. To their credit, my parents knew if they just gave in a little and gave us a slice—just one each—we would be satisfied and leave them to the rest. We also knew better than to push for more.

This unspoken arrangement became the accepted routine. One day, my parents forgot this little deal we made, and tried to hog the pizza all themselves.

It was a lovely summer evening. My brother and I had already been given our supper, and come to find out, mom and dad had ordered a pizza for theirs. They headed out to the picnic table in our backyard, with the entire pizza, to soak up the late day sun and share a quiet moment together. They didn't offer us a slice. Not even one little bite. We were left in the house with the lingering, intoxicating aroma of freshly cooked tomato sauce, melted cheese, and that warm, bready crust. Our mouths started watering. How could this be? Had they forgotten? We decided to help them remember.

Having already eaten had nothing to do with this. There's always room in the "pizza tube" as my brother would explain. Our bodies also contained "tubes" for dessert and other goodies, many of indeterminable size due to their apparent infinite capacity. (Conversely, the "vegetable tube" was very, very small.) We were always ready to see just how much the tasty food tubes could hold, but we felt we never really had the opportunity, except once perhaps. When my brother was in his late teens, he bought and ate an entire bag of Twizzlers and subsequently maxed out his "candy tube" as evidenced by the gobs of red-painted vomit coating our kitchen sink. (Indeed, not all research experiments end well, but much knowledge can be gained in the name of science.)

There they sat, indulging in the parents-only pizza. My brother shot me a look of determination.

"Here," he said. "Let's get some bread. We are going to eat it at the window and stare down at them as if we are poor starving children."

"Okay!" I agreed as I grabbed my own slice.

"No, no," he corrected. "We are going to share *one* piece. It has to look believable."

There we stood, in the spirit of true teamwork, Hansel and Gretel hunched together in the window like poster children from a third world country, hovering over one small crust of bread as if to protect it and us from some unforeseen element. Slowly and delicately, my brother tore off a little piece for me, and like field mice, we gingerly nibbled the tiny bits using both hands, while our Bambi eyes stared longingly at the bountiful feast of plenty our parents savored out back without us.

We figured our antics may not result in the acquisition of a slice of pizza, but we were going to make darn sure they felt horribly guilty about it. They made us drink all that veggie juice. This was a matter of fairness.

Mom and Dad tried to continue eating. They held out for several minutes. Somehow the feeling of small, desperate eyes watching keenly from afar drove them to the conclusion that they weren't going to enjoy the rest of their meal until they shared some of it with us.

They were right. And we got our pizza.

It's All about Access

In our family, Halloween was no joke. This was the one and only time of year my brother and I had hours of unsupervised access to pounds of sugar-laden, artificially colored, artificially flavored, chemically enhanced confections. More importantly, it was one of our limited opportunities to get our hands on a respectable amount of cold, hard, cash.

Instead of letting my brother and I pig out on all of these sweets (save the few bonbons we managed to stuff into our mouths while trick-or-treating), our parents *paid* us for what we gathered on Halloween, and then they did with it what they would. (Usually it headed to work and the break room goody-jar, or right back into the bowl to be handed out to other ghouls and goblins that night.) Where it went didn't really matter to my brother or to me. We were interested in lining our pockets with cash, not candy. Money could buy us what we wanted; our mercantile aspirations went far beyond the possession of a few fireballs.

This arrangement changed everything. Halloween was not about sporting snazzy costumes and hanging out with friends. This wasn't just a fun little pastime, a diversion, or a quaint little holiday to us. This was a business proposition. In a housing development with hundreds of prospective candy-givers, we had the potential to make some real money. There were approximately two hours of prime candy-acquisition time. To make the most of the evening, you had to think logistics.

Here's how it worked:

- Don't walk. Run, but do it carefully. As you travel in a straight line between yards (not up and down driveways to the street and back; there is no time for this), swing your candy tote in front of you to avoid booby traps (low fences or strings marking gardens and property lines).

- No masks. You can't see or breathe. Paint your face or forget it altogether. And think practical costuming—something warm and flexible (you are about to run a marathon in what feels like the dead of winter).

- Plan your route. Like spokes on a wagon wheel or a slice of pie, exploit houses in each "wedge" and then stop by home base at predetermined intervals to unload before heading back out.

- Use a pillowcase, not a pumpkin. Hollow plastic "decorations" may have had the strength, but not the capacity to hold the sheer volume of sweets we lugged around. (Forget plastic bags—they're practically useless.) Maximize the time for trick-or-treating by keeping return trips to home base at a minimum. Pillowcases are durable and hold all you can carry.

- Houses that only hand out one tootsie roll (a *handful* wasn't worth more than a nickel) aren't worth it. Skip that house and head straight to the next.

- No sissies allowed. Out of breath? Too bad. Keep going or get left behind. (Kind of a scary thought on Halloween, really.) Thirsty? Need to go to the bathroom? You better do it before the sun goes down and the pumpkins are lit.

- Don't head in early. At the end of day, folks are tired. Catch them at the right time—just before the porch light goes off—and they are likely to dump the rest of their candy bowl right into your bag. If you are lucky, just one house a year will fall into this category, usually around 8 o'clock on a weeknight, but closer to 8:30 or even 9 o'clock on a weekend.

- Keep records. Remember which house gave out the best candy and plan next year's trip accordingly. Make the most of these chances for a better bounty by hitting up these residences early in the evening.

- You are never too old to trick-or-treat. Perhaps I shouldn't admit this, but I was still trick-or-treating when I was, well, much older than I should have been for such an activity, and was renting my own place. Dad handed out my candy while I went out fetching more with some actual children. Then, I simply recycled my bag into the bowl of goodies I was handing out. When you get nearly 280 costumed cuties at your address every Halloween (and you are a college kid on a tight budget), the supplemental candy helped subsidize my yearly financial commitment.

Money can motivate, so it's no surprise that young, smart trick-or-treaters saved piles of goodies to sell at school months after Halloween was over. Sugar-deprived kids who had exhausted their stashes weeks before now stimulated a lucrative candy market. Their high demand pushed up selling prices to amounts far exceeding the cash we could get from our folks for the same merchandise.

Cash kept us away from the majority of junk at Halloween, but the sheer quantity we acquired would ensure that some of it would make it undetected into our possession, and we still looked for opportunities to get our mitts on candy the rest of the year, too. My brother was ingenious enough to cut a slit in a clear, unopened, pre-Halloween candy bag, take a lolly or two, and then use see-through tape to seal up the seam, which was almost undetectable to a discerning parental eye, as long as he wasn't too greedy.

We learned how to walk down a hallway, or a flight of steps, and miss every creak, and then quietly take a cookie from a glass jar, rolling the lid back down so as not to make it clink. This was the stuff of experts.

So what does any of this have to do with juicing vegetables?

Quite a lot, actually. No matter how protected children are, they somehow find a way to get a hold of food that isn't good for them. There will always be holidays celebrated with sweets. There will always be birthday parties, brightly colored displays of confections located conveniently at kid-level in grocery store checkout lanes, and the great lucrative candy trade on the afternoon school-bus ride home. Junk food is easy for kids to get a hold of. Either they know where to get it, or they know a friend who can get it for them. It's practically inevitable. Smart parents should expect this, allow for it, and enjoy the ride. Handing your child a glass of freshly made vegetable juice several times a week is a form of "nutritional insurance." This phrase coined by Roger J. Williams, Ph.D., discoverer of pantothenic acid (vitamin B_5), reminds us to hedge our bets and invest in good health. In the next chapter, we'll talk more about why investing in nutritional insurance is so important.

It's all about access. Kids certainly have access to junk; why not be sure they have access to good food too?

GARDEN VEGGIE PRODUCE FOR JUICE

As far as my brother and I were concerned, it was indentured servitude. There we were, at least three days a week, shoulder deep in tangled vines, prickly leaves, and colonies of insects in our enormous backyard vegetable garden.

Dad took full advantage of the eighth of an acre of land our little house sat upon, and he stretched our garden from property line to property line. A believer in organic farming, it did not in the least resemble a neatly plowed field with rolling hillocks of tended soil, clearly defined lines of uniform seedlings, and not a weed in sight. Our garden may have had rows, but weeds and grasses demanded the same freedom to grow as the plants Dad wanted to cultivate. On occasion, he'd pull the weeds, let them dry in the sun, and then replace them as mulch around the vegetable plants or to line the "paths" between the rows. Breathing room was created around each of the desirable plants so they could receive proper sunshine and rain, but any space without precious plant cargo was free to turn to wilderness. Perhaps using weeds as mulch made economic and environmental sense, but to my brother and me, it looked terrible. Freshly tilled in the spring, our garden was clear of any vegetation and we all felt a renewed sense of hope that this was the year it would not look overgrown. Our optimism lasted a matter of weeks. Inevitably, the weeds would return. Soon, all kinds of plant-life peeked out of the soil, and all creatures great and small moved into their new habitat.

Kids are always embarrassed about their parents for one reason or another. We were embarrassed about everything and that includes the lawn. My brother and I would glance longingly at the properties to our left and right and the simple, practical appearance of their outdoor living space containing merely mowed grass. Over time, each neighbor decided to put in a small, well-groomed veggie patch. They were neat and tidy: there were cages and strings supporting each individual tomato plant in its glory; there were beautiful raised beds reinforced by lumber; and there were things growing that we thought we would have actually wanted to eat. The neighbors didn't have families of mice making homes in their heaping, steaming compost pile. The neighbors didn't have hoards of birds seeking refuge in their primeval landscape. The neighbors had magazine-quality, photo-ready gardens . . . and tall hedges that blocked their view of ours.

None of our friends had to work in a garden. Even if they had, it would have taken a few minutes to pick the cucumber or two for that evening's salad. The sheer inequity of it all was obvious. We felt unjustly oppressed, like sharecroppers on our own land. Our motivation to finish our work was simple: we couldn't play until we were done toiling in the hot sun. We tried to get our friends to help out by explaining that we'd be done so much *sooner* with a few extra hands. No amount of Tom Sawyer's technique ever got them to help. They found other kids to play with who didn't have to work for a living.

Come now, you say. Was it really *that* bad? So, you had to help in the garden. Big deal. You had to work a little. In return you got to harvest fresh, wholesome food.

Teamwork or Indentured Servitude?

Sure, there was lots of fresh, wholesome food. There were, amidst the jungle of weeds, rows upon rows of green beans, summer squash, zucchini, broccoli, cherry tomatoes, lettuce, spinach, carrots, cabbage, beets, radishes, onions, and the occasional sunflower. A reader might picture a lovely little sunbonnet-clad blondie with her nose in a mass of sweet pea flowers, but let me assure you—this was not the scene in our backyard plantation.

For a nine-year-old, serfdom was a hot, tiresome, looming chore destined to take away countless hours of summer free time. It was a sticky, itchy, dirty job that bore under our fingernails and turned our arms green. It was the sheer quantity of produce that had to be harvested that caused the most trouble. We would pick unripened tomatoes in five-gallon buckets. If you left the green ones on the vine to ripen in the sun, they usually would split open and rot. So we picked them green, and bucket after bucket lined our dining room walls. The days that weren't spent with our backs bending in the garden were spent with our backs bending over the buckets, pawing through them to sort out the ripe, ready-to-eat tomatoes, and the almost-ready orange ones from the green ones. It was rough on the senses. There were always some red ones we missed the last time that would be deep in the pail, squished, moldy, and smelly. Some you'd grab thinking you had spotted a perfect red globe, only to find it bursting apart between your fingers. These had to be picked out one by one and composted. Our compost pile, tilled into the garden soil each season, became the mother of all future tomato plants. (My parents did purchase tomato seeds, but only once.) An abundance of fresh, sweet bite-size tomatoes sounds lovely indeed, but there is something about mass-produced food that takes the romance out of it all. Most of the tomatoes found their way into the blender or juicer and were pureed as a base for soups and sauces. Much of this food was frozen and then reintroduced during the long winter months. Tomatoes were our constant companions.

The garden menagerie was home to many creatures, hidden discretely and just waiting for a small child to turn over the right leaf and scream to high heaven. My brother and I knew we were never alone. I, for one, was terrified of spiders. My dad would point out that they acted as natural insecticides and helped kept plants clear of the real pests that would munch through our bounty. While I was okay with having fewer vegetables to pick and eat, Dad felt otherwise. Of course, this wasn't the only time we disagreed. For example, if I found one of these terrifying eight-legged creatures creeping around the house, I would simply murder it with the quick agility of a veteran assassin. If spiders weren't eliminated, they would find me. They always did. However, if Dad got to the arachnids first, he did not mush and flush as I would have wanted, but instead was sympathetic to their unjust persecution and *relocated* them to the garden as if they were part of some twisted witness protection program. They were there, all of them, in the garden and waiting for me, and I knew it.

My brother, on the other hand, was terrified of toads. I felt he was lucky to be afraid of something that generally inhabited the outdoors. He never had to wake up to one dangling in front of his sleepy face in the bathroom mirror. But, this fear made the trip down our concrete porch steps a harrowing adventure for him on a rainy school morning. And it made gardening positively horrific.

Our only savior was in fact each other. My brother didn't mind enormous spiders, and I didn't mind toads. While I was brave enough indoors to tackle a daddy longlegs head on with a roll of paper towels, the outdoor, hardy, fresh-air variety of spider that thrived on the all-you-can-eat bug buffet in our garden—and had the abdomen to prove it—were more than I could manage. These spiders were too huge and scary to be crushed by me (at that size they were practically human) and were to be dealt with for the agreed upon fee. My brother felt the same about amphibians, and so our arrangement prospered.

The going rate for removal was twenty-five cents per job. I don't think money ever exchanged hands for it was never long before the other would be called upon to pay his or her debt. Nevertheless, specific stipulations were put in place so the transaction could be considered legitimate. As per our toad-agreement: at a distance no less than twenty feet from the afflicted party (or better yet, the client could just wait indoors), the leathery skinned creature was to be placed in a high-sided drywall bucket; manually carried out to the far edge of the back field (an expanse that ensured no "incredible journeys" back to into our yard); and then dumped in an undisclosed location. On the other hand, the rules required that spider wrangling be carried out in the vicinity of the client to guarantee proper handling. The hired hand had the option of several methods of disposal. For instance, the spider could be swiftly dispatched with the sole of a shoe or—the humane option—it could be jarred in a clear vessel (to visually guarantee the presence of its contents) and capped with a tightly fitting lid to minimize the chance of escape, and let go in the back field, to join its toad friends. I imagine that a child or two that played back there in that field may have noticed a marked rise in two particular species of animals. For the most part however, the customer was not to be made aware of what was done with each culprit once it was removed from its original habitat. Such knowledge was an unnecessary burden for those wishing to distance themselves from the deed.

Somehow, no matter how many toads and spiders we removed from the property, more always found their way into the wildlife magnet that was our veggie patch. Our fears turned the boring, cumbersome task of gardening into a rollercoaster of adrenaline peaks as we just waited . . . waited for one of our nightmares to surface again.

It wasn't just scary for us. I'm pretty sure our parents wanted nothing to do with the terrors that lurked in that garden either. I never saw one of them take on a tomato worm without being armed with a shovel.

So, my brother and I sang lighthearted songs. It shifted our focus from our task and allowed the time pass more easily. (My grandfather would call this "whistling past the graveyard.") We were certain that instant classics such as "There's a Lima Bean in My Limousine" and "Oni-Oni Onion" were destined for the top-ten charts. When original music failed us, we switched to cinema and staged dramatic performances of *Big Guy and Little Girl* in which Big Guy would swoop in and rescue Little Girl from any number of scary situations, real or imagined.

Sometimes, no amount of creativity and teamwork kept us from the reality of our situation. Gardening was tiring and boring and hot, and then we had to eat the stuff too. I wasn't above stomping on a few zucchini flowers, but somehow shortages never occurred. We weren't going to get out of eating all this produce. So, we started to figure out ways in which we could get it over with faster. This is where the juicer came in handy: drinking our vegetables was easier. Piles of vegetables on our plates could be condensed into a few ounces of liquid in a glass. We would often marry zucchini with carrots to make a "Carrot-tini," which actually tasted pretty good. The zucchini mellowed out the carrot a bit and made it taste a bit lighter and thinner. My brother once asked for lettuce juice to avoid chewing a massive salad, but he never asked again. (I wouldn't recommend juicing lettuce, and neither would he, although my Dad would.)

Lessons Learned from the Garden

If you are keen on using a variety of fresh vegetables to juice, and you'd like the added benefits of knowing exactly where they come from and how they were raised, having your own garden may be just the thing, but don't expect your kids to have similar aspirations.

Gardening wasn't something we enjoyed. We envied the hassle-free lives of friends. We really thought the grass was greener on the other side of the hill. So, we went and got it.

Obtaining grass clippings became a business in our household. Dad wanted mulch, but prepackaged fertilizer was expensive. If you don't have a lot of money, and our family didn't, grass clippings can provide nourishment for plants as they break down as well as prevent weeds, protect the soil from drought, and keep the dirt around vegetable plants moist and cool on arid summer days, cutting back the need for constant watering. The amount of grass clippings Dad could obtain from our yard was limited, so he started to pay my brother and I for clippings we collected from houses throughout our neighborhood.

On Wednesdays each week, the streets would be lined with bags of lawn waste ready to be picked up for trash day. My brother and I would head out and gather as many clippings as we could before the garbage truck came by. We'd heft them into our red wagon, wheel them home, and collect between ten and twenty cents per bag, depending on weight. It was our job to see that the clippings were clean. The contents of the bag had to be free on any trash, dog droppings, or other lawn debris, so we'd open and inspect them for purity before making the journey back. If there was anything but grass in the bag, we'd go right up and knock at the door. By mentioning what we were up to, over time, many families would set aside clean clippings for us to pick up making our job even easier. Some might say that lawn clippings contain pesticides and fertilizers and therefore would not be the best addition to an organic garden. While that is a good point, we found the benefits outweighed the risks. Purists could choose to go buy organic hay or straw instead.

Money can sweeten up just about any deal, and my brother and I were not immune to its charms. Collecting clippings, and getting paid for it, gave us a small sense of ownership in the garden. It served as a small reward for the long hours of servitude. As the neighbors caught on to what we were doing with all those clippings, an interesting trend began. Grass clippings were disappearing from the curbside as folks up and down our street were using them to mulch their own gardens.

Many of the lessons of gardening were lost on us at the time, but now can be observed with more clarity. We learned where our food came from. We worked hard to get it. We saw crops thrive and fail. We learned when each vegetable was in season. We learned how to live greener by composting kitchen scraps—raw vegetable peelings, egg shells, even coffee grounds and tea bags. Usually bound for landfills, instead this "waste" turned our bare, topsoil-scraped clay land into twelve inches of lush earth. We learned that all it took was a little packet of seeds, a fertile pile of compost, a patch of earth, and some hard work to grow our own food. We learned about using spiders as natural bug-killers, grass clippings as free mulch, and how to pick and prepare what we ate. We learned that juicing vegetables was a quick, effective way to get nourishment from large quantities of our harvest. And we learned how to be healthy, which was probably the best lesson of them all.

BEWARE: GARDENS LEAD TO HOUSE PETS

Most kids have normal pets: a cat from a pet store or a dog from a "puppies for sale" sign. At least most of our "normal" friends at school did.

On our block, kids collected all sorts of things, and most had heartbeats and the means to escape, which is exactly what we intended to prevent. A lot of our pets never cost a penny. Many were strays, hand-me-downs, and creatures we found outside. Occasionally, we'd splurge and invest a few dollars in some pet store Rodentia, but this was rare. It was far easier to talk our parents into "free."

We didn't limit our animal collecting to just the lap-size and leashed variety. We had gerbils and birds and rabbits and caterpillars and fire-flies and butterflies. We had four to five tanks of fish at a time with sunfish from the lake that lived long, healthy lives and spawned thousands of babies, or goldfish from the local carnival which lived a few weeks at best. We accumulated tadpoles (until they grew legs and Mom made us toss them back outside, to my brother's extreme relief), cray-fish, clams, zebra mussels (when Lake Ontario was more polluted than it is today—really), and turtles.

We had hamsters, too—several dozen of them, and at least a dozen cages, with some fur-balls temporarily housed in five-gallon drywall buckets out of reach of kitty cats until proper arrangements could be made. If the hamsters had all been male, having an adequate quantity of shelter would have been no trouble at all. The guys lived in one habitat and got along famously, sleeping together in a large furry heap, whereas the girls each demanded her own cage to roam free, lest she murder the intruders. Since we were the proud owners of many a lady, cage upon cage lined the walls of our downstairs, also my father's

"THAT POOR DOGGIE! THAT POOR KITTY! UH, YOUR GERBIL LIVED *HOW* LONG?"

Animal health and juices. Really? Yes. Well, sort of. Like pets the world over, from the very dawn of domestication, they get the leftovers. The leftover in this case refers to the pulp extracted by the juicer. Our dog ate a middle-quality dry dog food. (And no, I [AWS] will not discuss brands: read the labels, check your pocketbook, and decide for yourself.) I would mix our carrot pulp, left over from daily juicing, into her dog food. This twelve-year-old mutt never needed to go to the vet except to be spayed. She was never sick. She could outrun me on a bicycle. (Just to clarify: that would be me on the bicycle, the dog on foot. Feet.)

Additionally, our dog got 500 milligrams (mg) of vitamin C daily, a multiple vitamin, plus 300 mg of calcium as she was getting on in her years. I'd give her 200 IU of natural (d-alpha) vitamin E once or twice a week. She loved the C and E and would actually do tricks for them. Multiples are not as delicious to doggies. You stroke a dog's throat to get it to swallow the multiple and the calcium tablets. That, or hide them in a marshmallow or a small gob of peanut butter.

Our cat got the same food as the dog, carrot pulp and all. In my opinion, there is rather little essential difference (other than price) between cat and dog food. So they both got dog food. It is a lot of fun to put identical food in the dog dish and the cat dish, and watch them switch and eat out of each other's bowl. They are sure that the other's food is tastier than theirs. Not in this house, mate.

Getting a cat to swallow a tablet is impractical to say the least, so we'd sprinkle a couple of hundred mg of vitamin C powder on top of the kitty's food. She had to eat through it that way, and does. Raw or lightly cooked egg yolk is another effective vitamin delivery device for both canines and felines.

Our gerbil ate raw sprouts and lived six and a half years. If you can top that record for an animal with 300 heartbeats per minute, please do.

Our pets never had an ear infection and never had a vet visit.

Yes, you too can make your pet a health nut. If the animal rejects the good food you offer, fast it for a day or two. Even so-called finicky cats quickly cave in. Remember, we are not trying to force unnatural diets on your four-legged friends. This is simply a way to get them to have more raw vegetable matter, nutrition, and fiber within the context and bowl of their regular diets.

office. Those seeking consultations with him would be inundated with
that light scent of pine shavings and the sounds of scampering, chewing, scratching, nesting, and playing. The click-click sound of rodents
sucking liquids from plastic water bottles with ball-bearing stoppers
echoed through our finished basement, and no doubt was a distraction
to his clients. But they came anyway. The only ones not welcome had
long tails and sharp teeth. This conspicuous buffet of tender, pre-
captured meat was too much for our kitties to bear, so we just kept
that door closed.

My mother, whom you might now picture as the most patient woman
on the planet, surprised even us when she failed to protest these newest
additions to the family unit: the wild mice from the garden that we
caught and kept. Most women would be dead-set on keeping mice out
of the house. Instead, these critters ended up at our extended-stay bed
and breakfast. My mother allowed them to be invited in, placed in fur-
nished apartments, fed until they couldn't eat another bite, and provided
with the daily human entertainment only our quirky off-kilter family
could provide. It was a pretty sweet deal, really, except the mice wanted
nothing to do with it. Invariably, overturning the soil of our garden in
the spring would unearth a few mouse mazes and send its occupants
scattering for new shelters. This made my brother and I feel badly. I
mean, we had just destroyed their homes. Shouldn't we replace them,
just like the insurance company would do? With sensitivity towards our
cause, and with a bucket handy, Dad scooped up the confused critters
and helped us move them to their new residences: cages in a place of
honor at the top of the stairs in our entryway. With unique, thoughtful,
inspired names such as Mouse-Mouse, the little brown field mice became
part of our family, at least temporarily. They spent most of their lives
cemented to the front cage bars gnawing the metal rungs in hopes of
obtaining their freedom. And while staring at their tiny, little, furry bel-
lies was fun, it wasn't long before we knew they needed to be released
back into the wild. Perhaps Mom knew their visit would be short lived.
I daresay she didn't miss the little fellas as my brother and I did.

Each year our garden provided a multitude of possible pet friends
just waiting to be made. If you happen to have kids who collect creatures and not just coins, at least now you can't say I didn't warn you.

"Don't You Dare Tell Your Mother"

Whether we liked it or not, every member of our household reaped the benefits of a high-fiber veggie juice diet: all of us. Yes, all of us. That means the cats and the dog, too.

Our pets often were rescued strays, drop-offs, charity cases from families who had to get rid of them, or as I mentioned they were the barn-raised variety advertised by a "free kittens" or "free puppies" sign posted along one of our country roads. The animals were always mighty happy to be taken in. I wonder now if they had truly known what their stomachs were in for when they took a ride home with the Sauls. Would the dogs have been so happy to hop in our vehicle, tongues lolling and tails wagging, to go home with us? Perhaps, knowing the alternative, the cats might have chosen to stay in their current environment and feast upon raw mouse meat, or whatever other tasty morsels they could scrounge up, weather permitting. But winter is tough around these parts, and our new pets were downright grateful for warm shelter and lively, loving company. Indeed, they had no place better to go. And neither, I might add, did my brother or I.

Many children would not be able to easily identify the thunderous sound of a 0.5 horsepower engine masticating many kilos of carrots. We knew it by heart. We could pick out that sound in our sleep, and it was often because we simply woke up to a breakfast of its making. So in tune we were with the juicer, we developed a sixth sense as to when its services would be enlisted. Predictably, every so many days, it would appear on the counter soon followed by the hum of whirring blades. This was a certainty if carrots happened to be on sale that week.

Chagrined, at our local IGA grocery store, my brother and I would follow several yards behind our father as he proudly strode through the checkout line and hefted forty-five pounds of carrots onto the counter. We prepared ourselves for a nosy grocery clerk who would, of course, be awed by the sheer volume of veggies weighing down her stand. Invariably, she would raise an eyebrow, look with disbelief, and then wonder, in all sincerity, what *were* we going to do with all of those carrots?

My brother and I were, of course, embarrassed.

Dad had many standard replies as to why he was purchasing so much orange produce. None of them made the situation any less mortifying. Apparently, we were the owners of several large horses, or just one extremely ravished one, dozens of bunnies, or, on occasion, an overgrown rabbit weighing more than both my brother and I combined, or any number and variety of goats, sheep, donkeys, or mules. The absurdity of the answer did nothing to alleviate the curiosity of the clerk. On subsequent shopping trips, the same question was always asked.

To make matters worse, we'd have to prepare the very food we didn't want to eat. The sink would be filled to the brim with carrots, and for twenty minutes, we'd scrub, scrub away.

Then, it was show time. There was no escape. There was no place to go. We knew we'd be handed a large colorful glass of pureed food. The juicer geared up, and the singing, song-making, and improvised dancing ensued.

"HA HA HA HA HAAAAAAAAAAAAAAAAH!!!!!!"

The banshee cry of my father did nothing to lighten our moods. What did is knowing we could have what we wanted to eat after we ate our "eligible food" (as my Grandma Saul defined as the food that must be consumed in advance of eating something far more delicious).

Enormous glasses were poured. "Scarf it!" Dad would declare, and we did. Then followed the statement: "Once you have this, then you can eat whatever you want, within reason." While chugging, we often thought of our reward. I was heading straight for a nice, normal bowl of cereal and milk. Mmm.

The juicer produced pulpy fiber-filled byproducts that my father deemed too nutritious to be composted. This carrot pulp was mixed with a measure of water, cooking broth, or other leftover food liquid, and a quantity of dog or cat food. We'd place this concoction at the feet of our furry friends, and they'd often look back as if to say, "Really?" Hungry and appreciative, they would eventually begin munching away, and promptly, as if on schedule, to the minute on the hour, the fiber would see its way into vibrant, orange lumps spotted about our backyard, so bright in color, they were quite easy to spot from some distance away. At our house, you don't eat the orange snow either.

It's true: the ratio of carrot to pet food had to be just perfect, otherwise they would rebel, hungry or not, and the carrot concoction would sit for hours, slowly drying and hardening until it crusted to the side of the metal bowl and took twenty minutes to dislodge with steel wool. It was a fine line, but Dad had it down to a science. Perhaps it was just coincidence that we never had a sick dog or cat on the premises. Not one ear infection. Perhaps their good health had nothing to do with the fresh raw veggies included with their dinner every so often. Our pets certainly never experienced an irregular bowel (although their bowel movements may have appeared irregular to a curious neighbor or two), nor did the human inhabitants of our household experience any irregularity, and if one did, it wasn't for long.

Generally, any food scraps or leftover liquids for the dog would be set aside in her dish and placed on the counter to avoid confusion.

Confusion?

Yes, because in our house what the dogs ate sometimes was what the people ate too; it was hard to tell the difference. For example, my father would often use stock for his soups and stews. The broth would be a combination of leftover cooking water from vegetables, canned foods, and pretty much anything else that was in the refrigerator vegetable bin or basket. Packed with nutrients that boiled off into the water, liquid like this made a perfect soup base. If there was too much fluid, the dog dish would get some. Once it hit the dog bowl, it was considered "dog water" and it would be used as a soak for dry kibble.

When the bowl was filled to the brim, it was way too much fluid for one pup's meal. Just once, I decided to save the rest for later in a pan that I set on the stove. I didn't think our good pan should be on the floor where the dog could get at it, but, looking back, I should not have left "dog water" on the stove where father could get at it.

When I returned to it to prepare her doggie dinner, I found my father cooking our dinner.

"Dad?" I said, looking at the pan he was using. Already knowing the answer I asked, "Where is the dog water?"

He looked at me a moment. Then he looked back at the soup he was preparing. Then back at me.

With a look that ensured I would keep my part of the bargain he said without missing a beat: "Don't you *dare* tell your mother."

Sigh.

I ate my meal with the rest of the family and without complaint. Heck, we let the dog lick our hands until there were webs of saliva between our fingers. (She was always very thorough.) Did we *always* wash them afterward? Some folks *kiss* their pets on the mouth. Did it really matter if our dog licked the bowl this liquid had been marinating in for a few hours? I tried to imagine that any dog germs were boiled and dead now. But then there was the mucus. I knew about doggie "mucoids." That's why we needed spatter-proof, two-tone semi-gloss paint around our living room and hallway. The top half was decorator-inspired matte-flat that beautifully diffused light; the bottom half was practical, easy-to-clean shiny paint. The trails of slobber virtually bounced off the lower walls. Weren't we clever?

Well, the soup tasted all right. There didn't appear to be any dog slobber in it, although I still couldn't help but wonder what mysterious particles were floating around in my meal that evening. At least my mom and brother had the good fortune of not knowing any better.

Events such as this did not slow anybody down. Juicing was a part of our lives and there was no denying it, except when I was out on my own and Dad wondered if I wanted a juicer for Christmas. For years, I said no. (I just knew he was aching to get me one.) Then, one year, I actually asked for one. And to my surprise, he gave me a substantial, durable machine that I still use today. My husband juices regularly and so do I. Even our baby girl gets CJ. (The cats have been spared, however.) Our family has personally experienced the health benefits that go hand in hand with a diet rich in vegetables.

I thought I would never touch the stuff once I was on my own, but instead it was just the opposite. Now we are doing it, too.

The folks at the grocery checkout are still mighty curious about all those carrots. And I know just how to respond.

CHUGGING A PINT IN FOUR SECONDS

Good judgment comes from experience, and experience comes from bad judgment. I guess that's why college was invented.

My dad often says that he raised his kids all the way until college without them having to take a single antibiotic. This is true.

The moment we got there though, all heck broke loose.

I'm quite sure I'm not the first kid to head off to university and discover what freedom really means. For the first time in my life, outside the confines of parental control, I was completely in charge of how I was going to live. It was a wonderful, liberating experience. I could go where I wanted to go. I could do what I wanted to do. I could eat what I wanted to eat. I didn't have to take my vitamins. Or drink vegetable juice. I had the freedom to *not* take care of myself if I wanted to. I could get sick, and unfortunately I did. I could take prescription antibiotics, and I did. I could learn that pharmaceuticals often don't work as well as eating right, vegetable juicing, and taking my vitamins. And I did. I had the freedom to stay up until the wee hours of the morning, party to my heart's content, and ignore, at least temporarily, how I had been raised. And I did.

Not all of my choices reeked of bad judgment; just some, and most of those were made freshman year. Decisions were made, both good and bad. I wanted to gain new experiences. From all of this, I defined myself, as many a college kid does.

One choice I made my freshman year was to get involved in team athletics. I never participated in high school sports, unless you count frantically whacking at a floor hockey puck (and the occasional shin) in gym class. I felt I had really missed out on something, and I wanted to make up for it.

Of course, I figured I'd start with a nice, friendly and uncompetitive, low-key, non-violent sport. I wasn't sure what that sport looked like. I didn't know how to play anything *at all*. I noticed that college club sport teams would often advertise around campus to recruit new members. When the sign hanging in the stairwell of my dorm said, "no experience required," it didn't matter that I had no idea what "women's rugby" was. I was simply thrilled that I qualified.

It turns out, I loved it. Perhaps best described as football without padding, rugby fulfilled my inner need to kick some occasional ass. It was an amazing stress-reducer. There's nothing quite like tackling somebody full force to make you feel just a bit better about life. Our team trained hard. We were good, too. We won often. It was fantastic. I was proud to wear my personalized rugby jacket around with my first name embroidered on the front. Opposite my name was the phrase "elegant violence" encircling a rugby ball decal. Anyone who gave me the once-over and a raised an eyebrow would be told no, this wasn't my boyfriend's jacket; it was mine. It was the only really cool sports gear I had ever owned, not counting my awesome spandex bike shorts, and I wanted full credit for it.

The girls on the team were a riot. They knew how to take full advantage of the college experience. The old phrase "the drinking team has a rugby problem" may or may not be true, and I'm not about prove or disprove that statement here. I can tell you, however, that I learned I could chug a pint of . . . um . . . apple juice in four seconds flat. (My brother is just about the only person I know who can drink a pint even faster—in just three seconds.)

I know full well where this "talent" came from. As children, when we were handed a large glass of juiced vegetables, often between sixteen and twenty ounces, we quickly discovered the best way to get it down was to do it as fast as possible. (Dad wasn't about to have us let any grass grow under the glass either.) And so, unbeknownst to me at the time, I learned how to chug down a drink. It was purely a matter of efficiency. And, to my father's dismay, I seamlessly transferred this knowledge into an arena where this ability was truly appreciated. I felt rather proud. My dad was rather chagrined.

Years later, I went back to visit my university. I decided to buy a pint glass at the college bookstore. It was a useful souvenir, and a sort of trophy I guess, if my talent was still worth bragging about.

Kids absorb a great deal about how they are raised. Much of what they learn does stick with them. Good advice occasionally sinks in. Family traditions and value systems shape who they are. Once children leave home, they may not always make the best choices, but somewhere along the line, because their family embraced good habits, that knowledge is accessible when they need it, even if their parents aren't right by their side. Maybe this is why parents muster the strength to let their kids venture off to college.

Having my own child makes this all too real to me. I hope to raise her with as many healthy habits as possible. She eats organic baby food; she takes a baby multivitamin and extra vitamin C; she drinks breast milk from a mother who juices, eats right, and takes her vitamins. My baby daughter watches me as I use the juicer, and she drinks carrot juice just like her mom. When she heads off to college, she may have an adult beverage or two, but I hope that she too will revisit all of the information her dad and I will impart to her about good nutrition.

Alma mater is Latin for "nourishing mother," which is exactly what the contents of my college drinking glass do for me. Instead of beer, the glass holds the pint of carrot juice I chug in the morning. Yes—in about four seconds.

4

———

HEALTH BENEFITS FROM JUICING

You can cure cancer; you can cure any disease;
or you can just maintain good health.
—CHARLOTTE GERSON, IN THE MOVIE *FOOD MATTERS*

"Good morning, class!" I (HSC) say with my biggest, most captivating today-is-a-wonderful-new-day voice.

"Good morning Mrs. Case," they reply, not half as energetically.

"Let's try that again . . . "

ENERGY

Teaching middle school is an awesome task. It is high energy, high stress, and also extremely rewarding. You get to be around kids that need you and crave your attention, and at the same time long to be independent and adult-like. It is a wonderful job if you can be very loving and very strict all at the same time, and don't take yourself (or their mood swings) too seriously.

First period classes are notoriously well behaved. The kids aren't particularly awake yet, which is probably why. The best way to get them energized is to come in bright-eyed and bushy-tailed yourself. A teacher's enthusiasm can be quite contagious.

One morning, I was discussing with my students the kind of breakfast they need to eat before a state exam (or any day for that matter) so they are alert and ready to think. Before they shared what they usually ate, I asked them first what they think I have for breakfast.

No takers.

I give them a hint and say it has the initials "CJ."

"Cranberry jelly and toast!"

"Cereal and juice!"

"I know!" pipes up a voice in back. "You have *carrot juice!* That's why you have so much energy!"

What an intelligent young lady. It's true: I almost always drank carrot juice before work. I found it easy to swallow—literally. You won't find me eating something dry and crumbly in the A.M. that turns to paste in my low-moisture morning mouth. My orange shake was also healthy. Loaded with beta-carotene, carrot juice is an immunity booster I really need before I go to hang out with a bunch of germ factories all day. (I've actually watched them use their quizzes as Kleenex.) Juicing in the morning is an easy routine to get into for me. Putting it off until later means it probably won't happen. My juicer lives on the counter, and

IF YOU CANNOT WOW THEM WITH WISDOM, BAFFLE THEM WITH BOTANY

When I (AWS) taught biology, one of the core concepts in the curriculum was plant photosynthesis. It still is, and always will be. That's because it is important, and, well, all life on Earth depends on it. Photosynthesis is just what the name implies: the word *photo* means "light" and y'all know what synthesis means. What the name does *not* tell you is exactly what the plant synthesizes with that light. The answer is: food. A green plant uses sunlight to make its own food out of water and carbon dioxide (the increasingly infamous greenhouse gas that our planet has too much of). So this waste gas not only provides food for itself, but also for us when we eat the plant or any delectable part of it. I would tell my slightly bored-by-botany students that if they did not think that "CO_2 plus H_2O yields $C_6H_{12}O_6$ and oxygen" was all that big a deal, then they should try doing it. "The smallest bit of green pond scum can make food and you can't," I'd say. "If you stand out in a sunny field all day, the only things you will synthesize are suntan and appetite." Plant power! We run on it.

it's assembled and ready to go in the morning. It takes only minutes (about ten to fifteen) to thrust some carrots into it, pour myself a glass and drink it, rinse the juicer parts, and mop up any mess, which is about as long as it would take me to prepare and eat any other breakfast, even if it's simply a bowl of cereal.

Juicing in the morning may be something worth trying, especially if "I don't have time for that" or "I'm too tired to juice when I get home" are part of your excuse arsenal. (See Chapter 7, Juicing Excuses, for others!) Getting it done in the morning gives you a sense of accomplishment all day. You've ingested a megadose of veggies that are super good for you. How awesome would it be to know that you've already eaten two pounds of carrots when most folks have just loaded up on sugar and starch? To those that would argue juice doesn't "stick with them," I would say neither does a bowl of Cheerios. Juice first. At least then it is done. Then, if you still need more to eat, add some protein to your diet now or a bit later—like an apple with a bit of peanut butter during your first break. To keep up our energy levels, we know we should probably be eating several small meals a day rather than having three large ones anyway, so make juice the first great-for-you food that goes into your body before work.

DIGESTIVE TROUBLES

In *The Vitamin Cure for Women's Health Problems,* I wrote a about a woman named Lydia and some intense gastric pain she was feeling after she ate. I wrote about how juicing cured her. Well, the secret is out. That woman was me.

It was awful. I can still remember the stabbing, gripping discomfort I would feel under my right rib, especially if the food I had just consumed contained fat or oil. Foods cooked in any amount of grease— even if they were just veggies—were a problem. A little butter on toast? Ouch. A chunk of cheese to nibble on? Forget it. To make matters worse, the pain was accompanied by nausea. Instead of spending my post-dinner time with my husband happily huddled up on the couch, I spent it hunched over the sink, worried that I was going to be introduced to my dinner again.

My doctor thought this intolerance to fatty foods might be due to my gallbladder. My grandmother had hers out; it was possible this was genetic. After a magnetic resonance imaging (MRI) scan, nothing was discovered. No stones. No abnormalities. Nothing weird at all. Everything appeared to be fine, but I was still in pain. It wasn't going away.

Stress rears its ugly head in many forms, and it was a likely contributor to my health complaint at the time. Stress-reduction activities helped, but I was still suffering after meals. I didn't have a label for what I was experiencing, but I wasn't about to sit around and wait for one either.

I knew about taking my vitamins—especially C and A, which are

CABBAGE JUICE:
THE OTHER "CJ"

Garnett Cheney, M.D., treated 100 *hospitalized* peptic ulcer patients with four glasses of raw cabbage juice every day. Relief from pain was rapid, as was total time to heal.

Said Dr. Cheney: "Relief of pain occurred in this series of cases without the continued use of any form of drug therapy and without frequent feedings of food . . . The rapidity of healing is emphasized when the average (cabbage juice) healing times of 14 days for gastric ulcer and 12.9 days for duodenal ulcer are compared with the 42 days and 37 days cited from the literature."[1]

In 1952, Dr. Cheney's findings were published in the journal *California Medicine.* The *Journal of the American Medical Association*[2] was not overly impressed, but Dr. Cheney's cured patients certainly were. There is further discussion of Dr. Cheney's work in my (AWS) book *Doctor Yourself,* where appears a longer account this interesting case story of a client I worked with.

Marjorie, age fifty-three, came to visit. She was losing half a cup of blood a day rectally. That is a lot of blood; a younger woman's entire five-day menstrual flow is only about that much. Marjorie was worried, and rightly so. She had seen an assortment of doctors, and was currently under the care of a proctologist who could find nothing really wrong with her bowel. He found some slight, general inflammation during a sigmoid-

both protective of tissues; I knew how to eat right—and I was actually doing it. But I couldn't even eat my favorite dressing on my huge dinner salads. Oil was oil and it hurt after I ate it. What I already knew about nutrition wasn't enough. I needed more information.

My dad told me about Garnett Cheney, M.D., a professor of medicine at Stanford University in the 1950s, and his ulcer patients. One hundred of his patients healed their peptic ulcers by drinking a quart of raw cabbage juice every day.[3] After a week's time, 81 percent of them suffered no symptoms. Success was also seen in patients with gastric ulcers and duodenal ulcers. There was something about cabbage juice, all right. Not sure exactly what to call it, Dr. Cheney referred to its healing property as "vitamin U" for want of a better title.

---

scope examination, but no lumps, bumps, polyps, or lesions of note. He told her that there was nothing to be done except to keep an eye on it.

Marjorie's question to me was the obvious one: "What can be done"? She was willing to try anything. My standard answer, and it is also the truth, is that I wasn't sure, but natural therapies were generally worth a full and fair trial.

Figuring that it would be hard to hurt yourself with cabbages, unless you dropped them on your toe or something, I told Marjorie about the study. She was a lot more interested than a healthy person would have been, and said she'd do it. She called back a week and a half later. She hadn't bought a juicer, but was putting fresh cabbage through her blender, and then straining it through cheesecloth to get the juice. She was drinking four glasses a day in this way. Her bleeding had been reduced to a teaspoon on most days, and no blood at all on others. She was delighted.

Then, the really odd part of the conversation began: she had been to her proctologist, and told him of the improvement. He was pleased, of course; nothing odd about that. She then asked him if he'd care to know what she'd been doing lately. Indeed he did, he claimed, adding that a doctor was always interested to know what helps his patients. So she said, "Do you really want to know"? He again said, "Yes." So she told him that she'd been drinking a quart of fresh, raw cabbage juice every day. He stared back at her for a long moment, and then said, "No, that couldn't be it." But it was. Marjorie knew for certain, because she is the one who did it.

I wasn't particularly excited about the idea of drinking glassfuls of liquefied cabbage. (Who would be?) But I was even less excited about my gastrointestinal pain. Mixed into other juice blends, I liked it just fine. But on its own? It sounded downright awful. On the other hand, it couldn't hurt anything but my pride. I guess could try to choke some down. After all, it was only one week of my life.

So, I went shopping for boatloads of cabbage. I can tell you I was the only gal in the place with a dozen heads of cabbage on the checkout counter. Incredibly, I wasn't assaulted with any questions about my purchase. That was fine with me. I didn't have a good answer prepared anyway.

I held my nose a lot that week and drank down sixteen ounces of my freshly juiced all-cabbage beverage twice a day for seven mornings and seven nights. Cabbage juice is thin, almost exactly like water, except it is light green in color and packs a pretty strong and spicy aftertaste. Before I let go of my nose, I would shove a piece of dark chocolate in my mouth and chew it up really well. Call it a chocolate chaser.

Was it all worth it? Well, after seven days the pain was gone—plain as that. No surgery was needed. No expensive pills. Just a little determination and a little cabbage. Okay, a whole lot of cabbage!

CONSTIPATION, CHOLESTEROL, HIGH BLOOD SUGAR, WEIGHT GAIN, AND MORE

It seems that vegetable juice is just one more problem with the American diet (insert sarcasm). Here's a ridiculous tidbit from the Mayo Clinic entitled: "Vegetable Juice: As Good as Whole Vegetables?"[4]

Here's the question:

"Is vegetable juice just as good as actual vegetables for meeting the number of recommended vegetable servings a day?"

And now the answer from a Mayo Clinic registered, licensed dietitian:

"Low-sodium vegetable juice can be an easy way to increase the amount of vegetables in your diet, but you shouldn't routinely use it to replace other types of vegetables. Most adults should get at least two to three cups of vegetables a day. . . . [V]egetable juice has plenty of vitamins and minerals, but it's lower in fiber than is a serving of

YOU WON'T SEE THESE WRAPS IN RESTAURANTS ANYTIME SOON

Take one or two broccoli leaves (or cabbage leaves, kale, or even leaf lettuce) and wrap them around each carrot that you juice. Send the wrapped carrot through pointy end first. This reduces clogging and improves the nutrient content of your juice. Taste? Better than you think. Fresh carrots are pretty sweet. Of course the smell of pulverized broccoli leaves is a bit of a jolt: sort of like a meadow after a rain, or the smell of new-mown hay. Personally, I do not mind it. You'd expect that by now, wouldn't you. Pull up a glass and join in the fun.

most whole vegetables. Without enough fiber in your diet, you may risk constipation, high cholesterol, high blood sugar, and weight gain."

First of all, adults are *not* getting two to three cups of vegetables a day. If you are drinking vegetable juice, even if it is (gasp!) instead of eating other vegetables, you are doing *far* better than most people in this country. We could debate what is the best way to get your vegetables. But we don't have an argument if we aren't even eating them in the first place. What is more important than the form they take is that we eat vegetables, period.

Secondly, the author herself admits that a person's veggie intake can include canned and cooked products. So why are we picking on vegetable juice? Homemade, fresh raw veggie juice sounds far more nutritious than any can of six-month-old peas. (But please, eat peas too!) And what if the vegetable juice is bought in a can? How come any other form of veggie is okay with her, but the juiced form "shouldn't routinely [be] use[d] to replace other types of vegetables"? (Are we back to that can of peas?) This doesn't make sense.

> TIME magazine ran a feature on Dr. Cheney's cabbage juice research in its January 1, 1945 issue, stating that "Tests on patients have been encouraging; their ulcers got better."

The author also suggests that drinking vegetable juice alone (and not eating whole vegetables) means you won't be ingesting enough fiber and this will increase your risk of constipation, high cholesterol, high blood sugar, and weight gain. She happens to be wrong, but we'll get to that in a minute. Folks, the lack of fiber in our diets isn't from drinking too much of that darned vegetable juice. It is because of all the other good-for-us food that we are *not* eating. A person who consumes more veggies, in any form, is going to be getting more fiber than those folks who don't make healthy eating a priority. Raw, homemade vegetable juice does indeed contain quite a lot of fiber, both soluble and insoluble. Soluble fiber is the kind that reduces "bad" low-density lipoprotein (LDL) cholesterol. Insoluble fiber is the kind that is good for your gut because it has a laxative effect and helps move material out of your gastrointestinal tract. The waste your juicer produces contains predominantly insoluble fiber, but that does not mean there is none in your beverage. Insoluble fiber will still make it into your glass. Still not convinced? Drink a pint or two of fresh, raw carrot juice and see what I mean. Your regularly scheduled, timely and comfortable bathroom visits will speak for themselves.

Is eating fresh, uncooked, fiber-rich whole vegetables a good idea? Sure! But so is drinking them. It goes something like this: if juicing gets you to consume more vegetables, and therefore more fiber, this is good. Juicing improves taste and absorption, which is also good. There's nothing wrong with liquid veggies. As far as I'm concerned, any advice that moves us away from eating vegetables is bad advice. Juicing encourages us to eat more of the very things we are not eating enough of.

CAROTENE COUNTING AND IMMUNE STRENGTHENING

Ideally, 6 milligrams (mg) of beta-carotene can be converted into about 10,000 international units (IU) of vitamin A in the body. The carotene in just one medium carrot could provide 5,000 IU of vitamin A.[5] There is some question as to just how efficiently everyone's body can actually make vitamin A from carotene, and theoretical yields are likely to be overly optimistic.

It takes me (AWS) about eight large carrots to make an eight-ounce glass of carrot juice using an inexpensive centrifugal juice extractor. (The yield from a quality masticating juicer is higher.) Since consider-

VEGETABLES: MOST OF US AREN'T GETTING NEARLY ENOUGH

Here's an excerpt from my (HSC) book *The Vitamin Cure for Women's Health Problems* that highlights the truly SAD (Standard American Diet) and the need for us to eat more vegetables. "Nutritional insurance" is a term used by Roger J. Williams, Ph.D. (1893–1988), who discovered pantothenic acid (vitamin B_5).

Nutritional insurance starts with eating more fruits and vegetables. Lots more, especially those that are rich in carotenoids, lycopenes, and antioxidants. Tomatoes, green vegetables like broccoli, carrots, cabbage, yams, and red, orange and yellow fruits—all are good choices. Government guidelines indicate that Americans should be getting five to nine servings or more of fruits and vegetables every day.[6] (Take it a step further, and make those *raw* fruits and veggies.) This really isn't all that much. Five servings measures out to be about two and a half cups of food or the equivalent of about one apple, twelve baby carrots, and four large strawberries.[7] Most of us don't even manage that. Only about 30 percent of us getting the recommended amount of either two servings of fruit *or* three servings of vegetables,[8] and only 11 percent of Americans are meeting U.S. Department of Agriculture (USDA) guidelines for both.[9] Surveys have found that there are a whopping 20 percent of folks out there that eat absolutely no veggies *at all*.[10] We don't even have to measure and count anymore. The USDA now recommends making half of your plate fruits and vegetables.[11] Look down and see what's there. A recommendation can't get much clearer than that. We must eat more of the right kinds of food; and when we eat more of the right stuff, we eat less of what we shouldn't. Our stomach is only so big! Eating a lot of fruits and vegetables can protect us against many cancers[12] and chronic diseases.[13] In fact, a higher intake of fruits and vegetables can cut your risk of cancer approximately in *half*.[14] That's pretty darn significant.

Sometimes what makes the most sense seems to be what folks rebel against. This is all too evident when looking at cancer patient research. The people that may be most in need of good food are probably not eating it. One study that looked at 9,105 cancer survivors and found only 15 to 19 percent were meeting the old five-a-day fruit and vegetable recommendation.[15] They are eating even worse than the rest of us. Perhaps there is a reason for the lack of healthy choices. Perhaps fresh fruits and vegetables are just too expensive. In a report from the USDA, a consumer could buy three servings of fruit and four servings of vegetables for an amount that is less than the cost of a candy bar.[16] Their suggested fruit and veggie budget measures out to be about 12 to 16 percent of a person's daily food expenditures, leaving well over 80 percent of the grocery budget for other foods, even in low-income households.[17] If that number is even close to accurate, then it's hard to argue that cost is the issue.

Okay, what about availability? Perhaps we just don't have access to healthy food. According to a 2009 report from the USDA, 2.2 percent of American households (without access to a car) live more than one mile from a supermarket and another 3.4 percent without car access live half a mile to a mile away.[18] This means that there are millions of folks out there who may not have easy access to nutritious food. But what about the other 95 percent of American households? What's their excuse? Apparently, even when access is improved, there is little to no change in consumption of healthy foods.[19]

So, it's not really about cost, and it's not really about access. What is far more likely is that we are just set in our dietary ways. Maybe we just choose not to eat what we know to be good for us. It's time for a change.

able pulp is discarded in the extraction process, the actual vitamin A content of a cup of carrot juice is certainly much less than 8 carrots times 5,000 IU each, or 40,000 IU. For most household juicers, I estimate it to be about half that amount. Juicers that conserve pulp will give you more. However, juicers that remove the most pulp deliver the best-looking, best-tasting juice. This is no lab exercise; a real person has to be willing to drink it. Therefore, for persnickety patients, do not hesitate to use an extractor.

Remember that liquefaction increases both the availability and absorptivity of the contents of a vegetable, while reducing the amount you have to chew. It is more an issue of quality than quantity. It is also easier and faster to down a glass or two of juice as compared with eating several trays full of produce. Furthermore, juicing avoids cooking, and natural health authorities universally recommend more raw foods in our diet. Remember also that carotene's vitamin A potential has little to do with its role as an antioxidant. For example, 20 mg of synthetic beta-carotene is inadequate to provide lung cancer protection, but several times that, in natural form, is protective.

In a 1985 study, carotene in high doses was specifically shown to strengthen the immune system by helping the body to build more helper T cells.[20] These are preeminent among your body's white corpuscles, that cellular National Guard that is the mainstay of your immune system. The amount used in this well-controlled study was 180 mg of beta-carotene per day. This is, theoretically at least, the equivalent of 300,000 IU of vitamin A per day! Were that amount consumed as preformed vitamin A (retinol), it would likely be toxic. As carotene, it is not. There is indeed a big difference between forms.

Incidentally, even AIDS patients have benefited from huge carotene dosages.[21]

Because the point comes up so often, may we repeat: excess carotene causes the skin to turn slightly orange. The medical name for this condition is *hypercarotenosis* or just *carotenosis*. *Hypercarotenemia* refers to elevated blood levels of carotene, and is also called just *carotenemia*. Both are harmless. According to the doctors' standard reference *Merck Manual*, "Excess intake of carotene does not cause hypervitaminosis A."[22] Hypervitaminosis A is vitamin A toxicity from the preformed oil

---

DON'T YOU EVER COOK *ANYTHING*?

Sure. Whatever needs cooking gets cooked. Potatoes, dry beans, bread, soup, rice, barley, oats, and more. Unless you have kitchen the size of a dollhouse, owning a juicer does not necessitate throwing out your stove. By the way, I (AWS) have no special expertise on cookware. However, I do not use aluminum cookware; I do not use non-stick cookware. Generally, then, this leaves the choice down to stainless steel or glass, both of which are well proven and inexpensive. Needing less cookware is even better. That means more "raw ware" (paring knife, cutting board, plate, juicer). If a food can be eaten raw, then it should be eaten raw. If it needs cooking, cook it.

ORGANIC: IS IT WORTH THE EXTRA MONEY?

"Yes," says Charlotte Gerson, "'Organic' is the key word. Carrots, for example, are used by farmers to 'clean' certain fields, because they act like sponges to absorb and concentrate poisons in the soil. So juicing non-organic carrots can even be harmful."

type of vitamin A, not carotene. Even with preformed vitamin A, says Merck, "recovery is spontaneous with no residual damage; no fatalities have been reported."[23]

In short, it is singularly difficult to kill yourself with carrots. Not only that, they may save your life. Literally.

CANCER

In the end, isn't this the one illness we're all really scared of? I (AWS) briefly discussed the Gerson therapy back in Chapter 1, and have discussed it more fully in my other books, including *Doctor Yourself, Fire Your Doctor!*, and *I Have Cancer: What Should I Do?* The most famous medical application of juicing is Gerson's protocol. The Gerson approach uses juices to nourish the whole body so the body will fight the cancer. It also uses juices to promote detoxification. Detoxification is a controversial subject. Heath nuts push it and the medical profession pans it. I submit that we put the matter to arbitration: you decide. Get into vegetable juicing and see how you feel. Or

> Albert Schweitzer's wife was cured by Dr. Gerson's vegetable juice therapy. Nobel Prize laureate Dr. Schweitzer himself called Gerson "a medical genius who walked among us."

read more about Dr. Gerson's juice-based cancer therapy on the websites listed at the end of this section and in the books listed in our Recommended Reading section at the end of this book.

The most common criticisms of the Gerson approach are that it is unsafe; it does not work; and if it did work, eating vegetables would do as much. These objections are without scientific basis. Vegetables, whether juiced or not, are safe. Do we really have to expand on that statement? Lincoln said, "I am weary of explanations explaining things explained." You simply cannot hurt yourself with produce.

As to whether it works, the books mentioned previously do a thorough job of demonstrating effectiveness. Dr. Gerson was curing many cases of cancer in the 1940s and 1950s. We also have recent research to confirm the effectiveness of his protocol.[24,25,26]

The Gerson Therapy

The lady who wrote the foreword to this book is arguably the greatest juicer on earth. At age ninety-one, Charlotte Gerson is also the longest surviving original patient of Dr. Gerson, as she was treated by her father . . . over seventy years ago. As we are rather obviously fans of father-daughter health teams, it is a special pleasure to see the Gerson therapy continue to gain acceptance and press worldwide. All this is primarily due to Charlotte. Her untiring educational outreach is the greatest possible honor to her father's work. I saw the results in my own clientele, and many people have seen videos of actual reunions of recovered Gerson patients of all ages . . . the majority of whom were once diagnosed "terminal." In addition to presenting Dr. Gerson's therapy, Charlotte has gone on record with some very strong words and absolute statements about pharmaceuticals and modern medicine. Here are some from personal communication I had with her in 2004:

> The chief obstacle to spreading this information worldwide is the powerful medical/pharmaceutical industry. Cancer treatments are bringing in hundreds of billions of dollars annually in the United States alone. The problem with the Gerson therapy is that it is not patentable, and produces no profits for the pharmaceutical industry. Therefore, they have powerful means, publicity, falsehoods that are spread by expensive TV and magazine ads to promote their "latest and promising" drug treatments. The general public is still convinced that only chemotherapy, surgery, and possibly radiation will help to overcome cancer. The advertisers do not publish the fact that each year the number of people dying of cancer increases, and more and more children suffer and die of cancer!

Only when all "orthodox" treatments have failed do some enlightened patients look for alternative treatments. That is why over 90 percent of patients coming to the Gerson therapy hospital are in "terminal" condition. If orthodox treatments could cure cancer, we would be out of business.

After my father presented five "cured hopeless cancer patients" before a U.S. Senate Committee in early July 1946, the medical establishment increased its attacks with articles in *JAMA* [*Journal of the American Medical Association*] on him. It published an editorial about the Gerson treatment with the heading "Of Fraud and Fables." It even either forced or paid a physician to retract his positive testimony during that hearing and had him write to U.S. universities and medical organizations stating that the Gerson therapy had no effect in the treatment of cancer! This letter was subsequently published all over the medical press, and reported to anybody inquiring from the AMA [*American Medical Association*] about the Gerson treatment. Other attacks were more subtle: Dr. Gerson stated that some 25 percent of his best cases were regularly contacted by their previous doctors, and asked to report on their progress. Then they were told that in their 'improved' condition, chemotherapy could now clear all cancer problems. When they agreed to take some chemotherapy, they died.

Dr. Gerson rented his office in a building originally supplied by grateful recovered patients. However, the staff (headed by the same physician I referred to earlier) spied on Gerson and reported names and addresses of his patients, many of whom were then contacted by their prior doctors and whose patients' files and records "disappeared." It was a fact that even at an advanced age (seventy-seven years), Dr. Gerson had low blood pressure and enjoyed one cup of coffee in the afternoon. He noted at one point that every evening, after having coffee served at his office, he had violent cramps and diarrhea. He stopped taking this coffee but a subsequent twenty-four-hour urine collection showed that he excreted arsenic! He did not die immediately; however, this weakened him considerably and he subsequently contracted a viral lung infection that killed him. Then, the doctors committed their ultimate insult: they claimed that he died of lung cancer! Of course his lung x-rays did not show tumors but lung damage from his infection. You will find a good deal of this information in my son Howard's biography of Dr. Gerson. Actually, Howard found it impossible to find a publisher in the United States. They were afraid of trouble from the AMA or "Big Pharma." The publisher in Canada who agreed to print the book removed about one-third of the stories that were highly unflattering to the AMA, the *JAMA,* and more.

Early memories of helping Dr. Gerson in the clinic would take us back to about 1949, in his clinic in upstate New York. My father's clinic was located in Nanuet, New York, just inland from Nyack. At the time it was a really small community but it has grown. I helped mainly by relieving him of having to do the daily liver injections. But it was more a learning experience making rounds with him. I remember a lady who had colon cancer with liver metastases, very ill, pale and bedfast. My father asked her at one point when she had had her last bowel movement. She was silent for a little while, so my father repeated the question. Then she replied, "I heard you doctor, and I am trying to remember. While hospitalized, I think my last bowel movement was at least six weeks ago!" I'll never forget my father's face on hearing this statement.

An interesting experience was that of a lady suffering from breast cancer. She was in an early stage, with "only" a tumor in her breast, still quite vigorous, eating and sleeping well and free of pain. But she presented a strange problem: she didn't respond to the treatment in any way, no better and no worse. And that was totally extraordinary. Then one day in the dining room, I overheard her talk to her daughter who was coming up to visit her from New York City. She told her daughter not to forget the salt to brush her teeth. That was a shock and I asked her if she brushed her teeth with salt. Yes, her dentist told her to do that. Of course, I told her to stop it immediately and also reported this to my father. I explained to her that the mucous membrane in the mouth is highly absorptive and that the salt goes rapidly into the body, encouraging new tumor growth. As soon as she stopped the salt, she had a normal healing reaction and was on her way to recovery.

After my father passed away, there was one overwhelming thought in my mind: I have to continue to publish his book A Can-

PHYSICIAN SUPPORT FOR GERSON THERAPY

The famous Canadian psychiatrist and researcher Abram Hoffer, M.D., Ph.D., editor-in-chief of the *Journal of Orthomolecular Medicine,* was a strong supporter of Dr. Gerson. Dr. Hoffer wrote:

> Max Gerson, M.D., treated a series of cancer patients with special (mostly vegetable juice) diets and with some nutrients including niacin (vitamin B$_3$) 50 mg, eight to ten times per day, dicalcium phosphate with vitamin D, vitamins A and D, and liver injections. He found that all the cancer cases were benefited in that they became healthier and in many cases the tumors regressed. In a subsequent report, Gerson elaborated on his diet. He now emphasized a high-potassium, low-sodium diet, vitamin C, niacin, brewer's yeast and Lugol's iodine. Right after the war [World War II], there was no ready supply of vitamins as there is today. I would consider the use of these nutrients in combination very original and enterprising. Dr. Gerson was the first physician to so emphasize such use.
>
> I am familiar with the Gerson method and believe that it has a lot of merit. I have always been frustrated that it was not taken seriously and studied intensively as it should be. It does take a great deal of dedication and time. Patients need a lot of help with obtaining organic food, preparation of juices, and other aspects of the treatment program. Of course, as with any treatment, not everyone recovers. But I think it has a very good track record. I know Charlotte personally and have been corresponding with her son, Howard Straus, who wrote a very good book about his grandfather called *Dr. Max Gerson: Healing the Hopeless.* I think it is a shame the National Cancer Institute refused to conduct adequate clinical studies, as the methods are not that difficult if carried on in a properly designed clinical unit.

cer Therapy: Results of Fifty Cases. I arranged for another printing and then had 3,000 copies on my hands. So, I had to sell them since they were not doing anybody any good stashed away in a warehouse. That is when I started to do health lectures in New York, first at the Foundation for the Advancement of Cancer Therapy, then for the various chapters of the International Association of Cancer Victors and Friends, and at meetings of the National Health Federation's many chapters.

One of my first lectures took place in San Angelo, Texas, during World War II, where my husband was stationed at the airfield. The various men's clubs were always looking for a speaker, and since a member of the armed forces is not permitted to address a meeting, I was invited. I spoke mainly about my father's life and my escape from the Nazis but, of course, couldn't avoid talking about health since it was an important part of my father's and my life. In all, I must have done hundreds of public lectures, also in Canada, Australia, Germany, England, Ireland, Austria, and Italy.

When we lived in France and I was only about thirteen or fourteen years old, we used to take a lot of Sunday walks through the woods from Sèvres to Versailles, visiting the castle and famous gardens as well as Malmaison. Actually, trying to think of my father's free time, he never took any. He almost never went to a movie, had no TV, didn't even go to the opera, which he loved. He was always working, reading, studying. I do remember just once when the whole family went to the opera in Paris. By the way, my favorite opera is still Verdi's Don Carlo.

> *I know of one patient who turned to Gerson therapy having been told she was suffering from terminal cancer and would not survive another course of chemotherapy. Happily, seven years later, she is alive and well. So it is vital that, rather than dismissing such experiences, we should further investigate the beneficial nature of these treatments.*
> —HRH PRINCE CHARLES, THE OBSERVER, JUNE 2004

I think that Prince Charles was very courageous to talk about the patient who recovered on the Gerson therapy. I also think it is horrifying and shocking to note the intensity of the criticisms—actually not criticisms but outright vicious attacks. Overall, it is amazing that so many of the "learned scientists" of the United Kingdom show such lack of respect for their crown prince along with lack of knowledge or interest in true healing. They never comment on the fact that the prince's acquaintance was terminal but recovered. And, that true scientists would jump on such a dramatic recovery and further study a treatment that obtained it. On the

Internet, even the title of the report on the article in The Observer is nasty: "Now Prince Charles talks about a coffee cure for cancer." As your readers well know, nobody ever claims that coffee is a cure, but the tone of the title implies 'See how this crazy character now talks some new nonsense! What foolishness will he commit next?' (Body-temperature coffee enemas are part of Dr. Gerson's protocol, depending on the patient.)

Then they [the scientists] talk about a "$20,000/year cost for injections on the Gerson therapy," which is simply not true. But what about the chemotherapy injections and their costs? The recently FDA-approved cancer drug, Erbitux, costs $2,400 for the weekly dose, or $125,000 per year, and although it has been shown to shrink tumors, it has not been shown to prolong lives.[27]

Internet Bias

Wikipedia's page about Max Gerson, M.D., is http://en.wikipedia.org/wiki/Max_Gerson. It is widely regarded as incomplete, untrustworthy, and lacking objectivity. A tally of approximately 1,000 Wikipedia user ratings (as of February 2013) averages about 1.5 on a scale of 5. Yet, the bias endures at this popular online "encyclopedia that anyone can edit." Gerson's principal biographer, grandson Howard Straus, tried to do so. Mr. Straus tells of some interesting experiences he has had with Wikipedia:

> Some years ago, on seeing that the pages for Dr. Max Gerson and the Gerson therapy were only stubs (short place-holders with little information on them), I put in all the information that I could, and kept it factual with references, citations, and literature links.
>
> Within a month, the following had happened:
>
> The information was labeled as "biased" and "unreliable" because I am Dr. Gerson's grandson and biographer. There appeared a big red flag at the top of the article labeling the articles, neutrality "dubious." The photograph I posted was removed. Provable, referenced facts, with dates and places, all suddenly became "claims." All my links, references, and citations were removed. They were replaced by links to the American Cancer Society and the National Cancer Institute, which offer only criticism of the Gerson therapy.

Even quotations from published scientific papers were removed. Attempts to rectify these actions were immediately overwritten.

It's easy enough to show the progression of the pages, since Wikipedia displays former edits on request, dated and documented. One can verify this by clicking on the "History" tab at the top of the Max Gerson page, and looking at 2005 and before. My editing is archived at http://en.wikipedia.org/wiki/Special:Contributions/ 69.109.140.164 and also at http://en.wikipedia.org/wiki/ Special: Contributions/Howard_Straus. A second Wikipedia page, specific to the Gerson therapy has been *completely* removed; see http://en .wikipedia.org/w/index.php?title=Gerson_therapy&redirect=no. To follow something of what happened, you can click the "History" tab here as well. ("The Hidden Wikipedia: How to Find Deleted Material about Nutritional Medicine." *Orthomolecular Medicine News Service,* May 11, 2010; available online at http://orthomole-cular.org/resources/omns/v06n18.shtml)

Reliable Online Sources about Dr. Gerson and His Therapy

- A review of the complete how-to-do-it Gerson therapy book at http://www.doctoryourself.com/gersontherapy.html.

- A transcript of a speech given by Dr. Gerson at http://www.doctor yourself.com/gersonspeech.html

- A review of Dr. Gerson's biography at http://www.doctoryourself .com/gersonbio.htm

- References and citations of published clinical studies showing the demonstrated benefits of the Gerson therapy at http://www.doctor yourself.com/bib_gerson_therapy.html and http://www.doctoryour self.com/bib_gerson.html.

- A review of *The Gerson Miracle,* a DVD about the Gerson therapy at http://www.doctoryourself.com/gersontherapy2.html, and a review of the 2006 documentary movie *Dying to Have Known* at http:// orthomolecular.org/library/jom/2006/pdf/2006-v21n04-p226.pdf or at http://www.doctoryourself.com/gersonmovie.html.

Also, see:

- Gerson, M. "Dietary Considerations in Malignant Neoplastic Disease: A Preliminary Report." *The Review of Gastroenterology* 12 (1945): 419-425.

- Gerson, M. "Effects of a Combined Dietary Regime on Patients with Malignant Tumors." *Experimental Medicine and Surgery* 7 (1949): 299–317.

- Hoffer, A. "Orthomolecular Oncology." In *Adjuvant Nutrition in Cancer Treatment* edited by P. Quillin and R. M. Williams. 1992 Symposium Proceedings. Arlington Heights, IL: Cancer Treatment Research Foundation and American College of Nutrition (1994): 331–362.

- The Gerson Institute's website: http://www.gerson.org.

VEGETABLES: GOOD FOR WHAT AILS *YOU!*

You may recall the story of *Aladdin and the Magic Lamp*. The magic lamp, the unprepossessing-looking, genie-filled lamp that Aladdin had, was old and battered. It was conned away from Aladdin by the bad guy, disguised as a vendor, as he called out "New lamps for old! New lamps for old!"

Not everything old is passé. If Grandma ate collard greens, turnip greens, dandelion greens, beet greens, lambsquarters (pigweed), or chard, don't dismiss her as an eccentric old fogey. If you, you-health-nut-you, enjoy big green salads, delight in the fact that they are absolutely loaded with minerals and vitamins. As my great uncle (AWS) often said, they're "good for what ails you." This is especially true when such foods are eaten fresh and uncooked.

A lot of garden greens get thrown away each year that could be eaten for better health. Weeds like lambsquarters, redroot, and dandelion are quite tasty when young and tender. When you thin out your beets or turnips, you can cook up the greens as you go. Raw Swiss chard, kale, or leaf lettuce is the basis a fine salad, and is simple to grow even in the smallest and most casual gardens. Any raw greens supply roughage (fiber) and many vitamins to your diet.

MOST CANCER PATIENTS EATING WRONG

This cannot be overstressed: *75 percent of all Americans do not even eat five servings a day of fruits or vegetables.* It is even worse with cancer patients. A study of over 9,000 survivors of six different types of cancer showed that only 15 to 19 percent were meeting the "5-A-Day" recommendation. That means that 81 to 85 percent were not. The researchers commented that these findings indicate that even a cancer diagnosis may fail to improve fruit and vegetable consumption.[28]

Better nutrition helps cancer patients live longer. This may seem too obvious to state, but its significance is still hidden from the people who most need to know it: the cancer patients themselves. Another study found that "the majority of new patients with cancer presenting to a medical oncologist are at risk of malnutrition or malnourished."[29] Specifically, 66 percent of patients were either at risk for malnutrition or malnourished. This means that two in every three new cancer patients are eating wrong. If there were ever a single argument for the vegetable juice-based Gerson therapy, this would be it.

I (HSC) spoke to a nurse recently who asked me what I would recommend for a cancer patient going through chemotherapy. I said, "Well, in addition to lots of vitamin C, buy a juicer and use it." To which she responded, "People undergoing chemo are not allowed to eat raw vegetables because of the risk of bacterial contamination and infection." She added that chemo patients are permitted thick-peeled fruits if the peel is removed. Thin-skinned fruits and veggies are forbidden. Wait just a hornswoggled minute. The very idea that cancer patients are getting the least of what they need the most is in itself sick.

Raw foods are especially good for your body. Raw foods and their enzymes have a definite effect on the digestive tract and the entire body's response to diet. The Swiss-German vegetarian Dr. Ralph Bircher, in an undated address in Wisconsin entitled "A Turning Point in Nutritional Science," said:

> There exists a reaction, which normally happens every time a person begins to eat; we call it the digestive leucocytosis. Some message sent by the palate to the marrow through the vegetative nerve system releases a deployment of leucocytes [white blood cells], which swarm out to the walls of the intestines, especially of

the colon, as if to defend a frontline . . . [Paul] Kouchakoff of Lausanne, [Switzerland] discovered that it does not happen whenever a meal consists of, or even begins with, raw vegetable food. This fact was confirmed by several other research workers. Then [Kaspar] Tropp [of] Würzburg, [Germany,] added another discovery. There are specific enzymes in fresh and living plant cells, which are very delicate. They perish when the plants are heated or even seriously wilted. They were thought, therefore, to be of no consequence to human health. But Tropp found out that this is not true. The human organism knows how to protect and escort these enzymes throughout the digestive tract, so that they can reach the colon without harm, and there they perform a basic change in the bacterial flora by attracting and binding what oxygen there is. Thus, they remove the aerobic condition, which is responsible for putrefaction, fermentations, dysbacteria and intestinal toxemia.[30]

Raw foods do not elicit the stockpiling of white blood cells in the digestive tissues, nor do raw foods signal the bone marrow to generate more of the white cells. This may be of the greatest significance to persons suffering from the disease, which *Webster's New Collegiate Dictionary* describes as "an acute or chronic disease in man and other warm-blooded animals characterized by an abnormal increase in the number of leukocytes in the tissues and often in the blood." The disease just described is leukemia.

Could leukemia possibly be a result of a diet of always-cooked foods? Naturopaths have long emphasized raw foods such as fresh fruits and vegetables, sprouted grains, and raw milk. If raw foods fail to stimulate the excess production of white blood cells, then perhaps an all-raw-foods diet should be insisted on in leukemia cases. From now on, when we hear talk of nature-cure therapies being successfully used against such diseases in other countries, we will see more clearly the basis for raw foods in them.

The enzymes that Dr. Bircher mentions as helpful to digestion and the prevention of intestinal toxemia fit right into the naturopathic approach to health. Pollution or toxemia throughout the body has its basis in the foods we eat and how we use them. Intestinal toxemia, abnormal colon bacteria populations (dysbacteria), constipation, and putrefaction from an overcooked starch and meat diet are all root causes of illness. In short, to prevent and cure illness, we therefore reduce meat consumption; increase our intake of whole, mostly raw foods; and (pretty much as an automatic result) clean out body wastes in the process. These are my "Three Quick Steps to Health." Raw food enzymes and the body's special response to them are a time-honored key to nature-cure.

In his address, Dr. Bircher cited a paper by the Swiss medical doctor Paul Kouchakoff (mentioned earlier) entitled "The Influence of Food Cooking on the Blood Formula of Man," which was presented in Paris at the First International Congress of Microbiology way back in 1930. If my references to early- to mid-twentieth-century research bug you, remember that Einstein's theory of relativity has held up pretty well, and that's not any more recent.

Read more, cook less, feel better!

JUICING: LET'S HEAR FROM PEOPLE WHO'VE TRIED IT

Here follow accounts of real people with varying problems who have been helped by juicing. Many did some juice fasting, which is a diet of fresh vegetable juices only for days or even a week or two at a time. Readers are also encouraged to look at Appendix 1 for more examples of people with cancer who have benefitted from juicing.

Boosts Mood and Energy

Sam writes:

I had already been taking vitamins, minerals, and supplements for neurotransmitter support, for a couple of weeks and my mood and energy are much better. However, those benefits seemed to fluctuate from day to day.

I read your article last week on vegetable juicing, and I've been juicing for four days now (and drinking water, but no solid foods at all), and I lost four pounds! Only sixty more pounds to go! I feel

incredible, all day, every day! I am a web developer and program-
mer, and I am amazed at how great the improvement is with my
memory, attention level, and focus. Plus, I can work all day without
taking a break, and I don't get stressed, like I used to.

I even have more energy to exercise now. It seemed counterpro-
ductive to exercise when I never felt good.

I can't believe how well the juicing is working, and it tastes
amazing. Plus, I don't really get hungry, but if I feel hungry, I just
drink more vegetable juice!

Cures Psoriasis

Rebecca says:

I just wanted to let you know I'm now free of psoriasis because
of you. I had had it from the age of eight all over my arms, legs,
and torso, everywhere from the neck down. It never went away or
faded from time to time; it was a permanent thing. The coal-tar
cream made it painful and caused it to bleed (and didn't help it at
all!) so I only used the stuff for a few months.

After reading your page on psoriasis, I juice-fasted. It started to
clear up in the first week and I was so excited! I wanted to continue
juicing until it was completely gone (rather than alternating with
raw) so I kept going and it took ten weeks to go altogether. My
skin at the end was unbelievable—so silky and beautiful. Since the
fast I've eaten a raw vegan diet, and the psoriasis has stayed away
(although my silkiness was temporary).

During the fast I found if I drank fruit juice, I felt better than
on just vegetable juice. It was mostly grape, apple, carrot or mixed
veggies.

I've also had what looked like a red mole on my shoulder since
I was eight. I can't remember exactly what it was called, but the
skin specialist said it was "second cousin to a wart." That faded
dramatically on the juice diet and is now barely visible.

I still can't quite believe that I have completely clear skin. It's
like a miracle. Whenever I read about someone with psoriasis in
a magazine or newspaper, I want to find them and say, "There *is*
a cure. You don't have to endure this for the rest of your life." I

want to shout it from the rooftops. Nobody should have to put up with it. I'm so grateful for your website, and for all the information you provide. Thank you for allowing me to feel comfortable in my own skin.

Lowers Cholesterol

Karen says:

My cholesterol numbers were through the roof. I was one of those people with very high cholesterol even though I ate hardly any animal products or fatty foods . . . and I was somewhat underweight. Apparently, my body was making it, and a lot of it: I was over 400. After two months of vegetable juicing, my cholesterol was cut to half that. No medication I ever took did what juicing did for me.

Sheds Unwanted Pounds

There are a lot of books on dieting, and this is not one of them. However, we'd like to point out that getting to your optimal weight is important, even if you only can pull it off temporarily. Yo-yo dieting is not ideal, but it is better than not dieting at all. Carrying a fat load is no joke: it is not called morbid obesity for nothing. Overweight kills. A mostly-vegetable-juice diet is better than any other weight loss plan we know. The best all around, long-term plan is eating right, exercising, and regular vegetable juicing. I (AWS) effortlessly lost twenty pounds juicing. Felt great, too.

THE PRICE IS RIGHT

If the cost of family juicing bugs you, consider this. The average baby goes through between 6,000 and 7,000 diapers before completing toilet training. Consider that at twenty cents per diaper, that's over $1,200, and diapers usually cost more than that. Get a juicer. You might just as well have a healthy baby as a dry baby.

By any standard of comparison, you can afford juicing. You have to eat anyway; you might as well eat what keeps you from having to spend time, money, and suffering being sick. I'm going to say it again, because parents need to know: "It can be done." My children were raised all the way into college without even one dose of any antibiotic. When we had insurance (which was rarely), it was delightfully irrelevant. Our kids had their physicals at school, and economically thus vetted, played outdoors, ate right, took vitamin supplements, and, by golly, drank fresh vegetable juice. Insurance did not pay for any of these measures that kept them well. Aside from physicals, there were no doctor visits. (I mean *none*; my son and daughter never even met their pediatricians.) No office call fees; no waiting room scream-a-thons; no co-pays; no medicines, prescription or otherwise. Such savings certainly covered the cost of the carrots.

5

MEGA-NUTRITION FROM VEGETABLES, THE FUN WAY

*The Learned Pig was a far greater object of admiration
to the English nation than ever was Sir Isaac Newton.*
—ROBERT SOUTHEY (1774–1843)

Not everybody sees the value in vegetable juicing. Some critics' egos let them forget the true healer's prime directive: "For the good of the patient, to the best of my ability." If there is a down side to vegetable juices, I (AWS) am yet to hear it. The worst reproach I've encountered is that, while harmless, vegetable juices have no special properties against cancer. How can that be, when doctors now know (and our grandmas have known for generations) that vegetables *do* in fact help prevent and arrest cancer. All vegetables are high fiber and low fat. Tomatoes are loaded with lycopene. Orange and green vegetables are tremendous sources of carotene. Broccoli, cauliflower, kale, Brussels sprouts and cabbage (the cruciform vegetables) are all heavyweights in the fight against cancer.

How, pray tell, could their juices *not* have anti-cancer properties? Juice consists of the entire cytoplasmic contents of a vegetable's cells, but without an unpalatable excess of indigestible fibrous cell wall. It's the corn without the can, the nut without the shell, the cash without the bank.

The two chief purposes of juicing are to increase the quantity of vegetables consumed, and to increase a patient's absorption of what is consumed. More vegetables is good. Better utilization is good. Ergo, juicing is good, and Dr. Gerson was right.

I find that, like a method actor, it helps to get into character before discussing juicing. To this end, I had two quarts of carrot juice for lunch and now I can feel the part in a big way. I am juiced up and in the groove. And for all my thirty years of juicing, for all the many miles on my juicers, I owe a personal debt of thanks to Dr. Gerson. He was pretty much the first physician ever to plainly set all this down into a clear-cut, specific therapeutic regimen. This is provided in great detail in his books.

WHY JUICE AT HOME?

You cannot buy freshly prepared vegetable juice in any store at any price—unless they literally juice the vegetables right in front of your eyes and you drink it down before they make you pay for it! Any juice in a carton, can, or bottle has been heat-treated and was certainly packaged at least a few days, if not weeks, months, or even years ago. This applies to frozen juice, too. So you need one essential and somewhat expensive appliance: your own juicer.

WHY LIQUIFY?

There is specific benefit to liquefying vegetables. Breast milk is a liquid.

"WHY JUICE? WHY NOT JUST EAT THE VEGETABLES?"

- Juicing means higher vegetable intake. You can guzzle more than you will chew. Juicing concentrates the good stuff and makes it possible to quickly down the goodness of five pounds of produce.
- Juicing means better absorption of nutrients.
- Juicing means raw.

Feedings for hospitalized patients are frequently in liquid form. The elderly often consume liquefied food. For the average person who is healthy and neither old nor infant, juicing still has proven benefits: *higher intake of raw vegetables and better absorption of nutrients.*

TYPES OF JUICERS

If you are looking for a brand recommendation here, you will be disappointed. We have no financial connection whatsoever with any juicer manufacturer, distributor, or retailer. And, we do not provide opinions on what kind of juicer you should buy, or where you might buy one.

Very generally speaking, there are four kinds of juicing appliances.

Blender

Yes, you could argue that a blender is not a juicer. However, some juicers are actually very powerful blenders. They yield a thoroughly pulverized but unseparated, unclarified product, more like a puree than a juice.

- Advantages: A total food, vast amounts of fiber, no waste.

- Disadvantages: Many people will reject even attempting to drink (slurp?) anything thick and unpalatable. The product may be pressed and effectively strained through cheesecloth. I know people who have done so, and I admire their moxie.

Centrifugal Juicer

This is the most common and popular type of juicer. Most cheap juicers are centrifugal, but not all centrifugal juicers are cheap. Many advertised-on-TV juicers are high-quality centrifugal products. Their disc-shaped blade rotates and shaves the vegetable, at the same time spinning out the fluid fraction. It is sort of like the spin cycle gone berserk on your automatic clothes washer. You tend to have wet pulp from all centrifugal juicers, and wet pulp means juice lost.

- Advantages: Low price, easy to use, not difficult to clean, fast.

- Disadvantages: Inefficient, blade assembly dulls quickly under hard-rock (e.g., carrot) vegetable use.

Masticating Juicer

This juicer has a rotating drum blade assembly that "chews" (shreds) vegetables into a pulp, which is then strained as it exits the juicer. You usually get a drier pulp, and consequently more juice from your produce with this type of juicer.

- Advantages: Efficient, long blade life (literally ten years or more in my experience).

- Disadvantages: Machine tends to generate more friction, and as a result it heats up, and, to some extent, the juice warms up. They typically cost more than most centrifugal juicers.

Grind-and-Press Juicer

This type of juicer presses the vegetables rather than spins or chews (masticates) a blade against them. Variants may also be known as manual, cold press, or hydraulic juicers. They are the most expensive type of juicer, some running over two grand. But, according to Charlotte Gerson, these are the best and the healthiest. She says, "As to the question, what kind of juicer? I heartily agree with Dr. Saul that the best one—for prevention—is one that you will use. However, for healing advanced pathologies, one should have the most efficient kind, which grinds and presses the vegetables." There is further discussion of this in the Gerson therapy books, listed in our Recommended Reading section.

- Advantages: Machine temperature tends to stay low so juice temperature is less likely to increase. Less heat is a good thing: it means less likelihood of food enzyme destruction. There are varying opinions on exactly how hot juice would have to get to destroy enzymes. The temperature would likely have to get to at least 120 to 130°F (and probably much hotter) for this to occur. That is pretty warm, the temperature of a medium-rare cooked steak. No juicer of any kind that I have ever used, no matter how cheap, even approaches that kind of heat. Nevertheless, the Gerson Institute specifies this kind of juicer, based on their clinical success.

- Disadvantages: Grind and press juicers are usually the most expensive, and most labor intensive.

The Bottom Line

My mother said, and often: "you can only spend your money in one place." May I add to that: use your money wisely: invest in wellness. It is cheaper in the long run. Spend as much money as you can afford to. Generally speaking, you get exactly what you pay for.

A true juicer is not a blender. A juicer makes juice; a blender makes raw baby food. There is nothing wrong with blending your foods. If you found such food to your liking, it would actually be very digestible. However, to make palatable juice you need to extract the fluid part of the vegetable along with the vitamins, minerals, and enzymes it contains. Therefore, you need a juice extractor. And we are not referring to a whirl-top orange juicer, either.

Be sure to get a really good juicer. Good juicers make tastier juices, faster. Good juicers also clean up more quickly than cheap juicers. We do not sell juicers. What we do is recommend that you get one and use it. A lot. If you have one, dust it off and use it. A lot. Bottom line: buy the best you can on the budget you have. In daily, practical terms, "the best" is the one you will *use,* and the one you will use is the one that *cleans up easily.* Later in the chapter is a section on how to streamline the process.

WHAT TO JUICE

You can juice almost anything you can eat raw. Vegetables are best, especially carrots, cucumbers, beets, tomatoes, zucchini squash, romaine lettuce, celery, and cabbage. You may juice fruits also, naturally. Freshly made raw apple, grape, and melon juices are delicious. It is not generally a good idea to juice potatoes, eggplant, or lima beans (not that you'd want to). It is wise to peel vegetables that have been sprayed or waxed. Sprayed fruits are also good to peel before juicing. Carrots and other underground vegetables often do not need peeling. Instead, give them a good scrubbing with a nylon-bristle vegetable brush while rinsing under tap water. Beets are the exception. Since beet skins are very bitter, it is wise to peel beets before juicing. A hint to save time: dip the beets for about 20 seconds in boiling water and then peel them . . . it's much easier.

Your juice will taste the best if you drink it right after preparing it. I mean within moments! Fresh juice contains a great amount of raw food enzymes and vitamins, many of which are easily lost as the juice sits. So don't let it sit! Drink it right down, with the thought that this is unbelievably good for you.

Combining Fruits and Vegetables?

Why, *sointenly!* First reason: taste.

Fruits are sweet, and generally too intensely so to consider as much more than juiced desserts. However, it is an old trick to improve the appeal of vegetable juices by adding some fruit to the mix. Not an issue with carrots: they are sweet to begin with. But cabbage and broccoli? These major-league flavors often benefit from a few grapes, an apple, or pretty much anything else that is in your fruit basket.

If you have heard it said that "you cannot combine fruits and vegetables," read on.

Second reason: botany.

Botanically, any seed-bearing structure that proceeds from a flower is a fruit. This means tomatoes are fruits. It also means that cucumbers, green peppers, green beans, eggplant, summer squash (yellow, zucchini), winter squash (acorn, butternut, Hubbard), and pumpkins are all fruits. Pickles are fruits, as they are cucumbers. Tomato ketchup (catsup) is a fruit sauce, and so too is pizza sauce. Pumpkin pie is a fruit pie, and sausage with peppers is actually sausage with fruit. Green bean casserole is a fruit casserole (and the mushrooms in the canned soup atop it are a fungus). So, to us it seems pretty silly to worry about combining any of these good foods with other "conventional" fruits.

The following vegetables are highly nutritious and among our favorites.

Beet Feats

If you think carrot juice is weird, just try to get folks to drink beet juice. A man with leukemia did. His wife and I discussed the benefits and safety of juicing vegetables, and I mentioned that beets have a long folklore of being good for the blood. This "doctrine of similars" (such as kidney beans being good for the kidneys) has long been generally discounted or dismissed outright. But there is such a thing as serendipity, and there is such a thing as benefit from folk remedies. One or the other of these factors worked for him. He did not willingly juice beets and drink them. His improvement was largely due to his devoted and energetic wife who, not taking "Hell, no!" for an answer, followed her husband around the house until he drank his glass of beet juice, several times daily. He hated it. She did not care if he hated it; she was out to save his life. His improvement was so dramatic that his oncologist literally came out into the waiting room and waved about his test results for the other patients to see. (This was years ago, and obviously before the Health Insurance Portability and Accountability Act [HIPAA], the privacy rule that protects patient's health information.) Beets were known to be beneficial for centuries before that. Put it all together and you have a man with physician-confirmed, laboratory-documented improvement. Not bad for beets.

But *was* it the beets?

One review[1] of the subject has stated:

> Beetroot has unique chemicals such as betalains [which] act as antioxidants. The therapeutic use of beetroot in cancer treatment came to prominence with the work of the Hungarian physician Alexander Ferenczi (Csorna, Hungary) in the 1950s. He introduced a revolutionary new treatment for cancer using nothing but raw beetroot juice. In his papers from the late 1950s and early 1960s,

he reported remarkable success in treating cancer patients . . . Ferenczi's treatment was based on consuming a liter of beetroot juice daily, for at least two to three months.

The reviewer also cites nearly a dozen studies on the wide-ranging effects and properties found in beets.[2] And then, there is Dr. Ferenczi's 1961 original paper: "Tumor Treatment with Red Beets and Anthocyans, Respectively."[3] Why would a doctor of medicine use this treatment and report benefits if there were nothing to report?

Behold the beet. Using a sharp, heavy knife, like a cleaver, carefully cut one open and prepare to be dazzled: a gorgeous, random yet elegant pattern of reds awaits you. Beauty and the beet! Those colors are due to the betalains mentioned above. When your awe subsides, it is now time to point out that you have to peel a good many of them to make beet juice. Why bother? "Beets? Bleech!" we hear avid *Mad* magazine fans chanting. But wait: there are more beety benefits.

Beets contain betaine (trimethylglycine), an amino acid with three methyl (single-carbon) groups stuck on it. Some athletes use betaine for bodybuilding and/or athletic performance-enhancement. Beets are considered medicinal by herbalists who regard beet betaine as a tonic, detoxifier, and liver purifier. Betaine is known to lower cholesterol and homocysteine levels, thus reducing the risk of cardiovascular disease. And, betaine also increases the body's available S-adenosylmethionine (SAMe), which helps to relieve depression.[4] Some feel that these attributes make it desirable for people to gradually increase their beet intake. I have been juicing for decades and have never known of a person suffering from beet overdose. It is singularly difficult to kill yourself with produce. It is certain that beetroots are a very good source of carbohydrates, potassium, trace minerals, several B vitamins, and vitamin C. Beet tops (which can be cooked up just like spinach) are a very good source of vitamin A and iron, as well as calcium and magnesium.

Here is entirely too much good nutrition to go to waste.

Speaking of waste, the first time you have any appreciable quantity of beets or beet juice, you are in for a surprise. Well, I certainly was. High-beet consumption can be relied on to turn bowel movements red, and sometimes even the urine as well. One otherwise calm and average visit to the littlest room in the house resulted in my turning about to flush and seeing a flash of red below me. The toilet water was red. I instantly thought, "Good grief: I must have the largest and most severe hemorrhoids in the solar system. I am hemorrhaging and going to die." And then I remembered I had consumed a lot of beets just long ago to have forgotten . . . until then, of course.

You cannot put all your trust in toilets. So take it from those of us who have, er, been there: beets have a strong, natural red coloring. Relax, it's just vegetables. Be aware but be calm. Remember to wash your hands. And speaking of hands, when you prepare beets, you will get nicely purple-dyed hands, rather like the racially conscious Petries experienced on the *Dick Van Dyke Show*. I have "beet hands" as I write this, since I downed a quart and a half of straight beet juice before sitting down at the computer. But you'd expect that, wouldn't you? The color wears off within a day.

BEET TREAT

My daughter and coauthor cannot make an "I have beet hands" statement. Nyah-nyah! Actually, it is my fault: I fed my kids one bowl of borscht too many when they were growing up, and neither of them will go near a beet now without an armed military escort. There is one exception: beet juice is a wonderful, natural red food dye. My daughter capitalized on this property to make the lovely and additive-free pink icing for her child's first birthday cake. The icing had no beety flavor whatsoever.

Gee whiz! While we are on quaint topics, let's talk about urine, shall we? Colored urine can mean something or nothing. Blood in the urine is obviously a see-the-doctor-immediately matter. But if you just drank nearly two quarts of beet juice, as I do and just did, your urine may be a bit off color. Not red, but to the reddish side of orange. This means that it contains the natural beet color, which is due to flavones. These colors are very good for you, and have anti-cancer properties.[5] Urine is filtered from the blood. The only way something can get into your urine is if it was in your bloodstream first. To be in your bloodstream means that you absorbed it thoroughly, and it circulated throughout your body.

"OH, NO! BETA!"

Even the recidivist criminal character Snake on *The Simpsons* would agree that beets look unappetizing and the color is weird. Some people cannot stand the smell of them. Even the scientific name for a beet is gross: *Beta vulgaris.* Well, you can blame the name on Linnaeus, back in 1753 when beets were first catalogued. But beets have been food literally for ages, dating at least to the ancient Greeks and Aristotle. Our common red table beet is known as *remolacha* in Spanish and *betterave* in French. The Italian, *barba-bietola,* sounds like a fashion-model doll convention, at least to me. But then, I have grandchildren.

Okay, now for the good part: beets taste great raw and juiced. Fresh organic beets taste best. These are the very unlovable-looking roots that I haul out of my garden by the bucketful. Why? Because beets are easy to grow. They are darn near bulletproof. You can, and should, plant them as soon as the soil can be worked. Even when there is still snow on the ground, or frosts every night, most will still come up. I learned hardscrabble subsistence gardening in Vermont, and the season is mighty short up there. Old-timers showed me how to get the jump on the season by planting hardy crops *really* early. Germination percentage for beets can be disappointing until you get used to it. Hint: do not plant them too deep or too shallow, but if you have to make a mistake, plant them too shallow. I have had beets grow literally on top of the soil, with only their tap root extension beneath ground. If they seem unstable (wobbly or prone to topple over), or they simply look gauche to you, add soil later around them as desired.

Here's the big beet surprise: beets are sweet. Indeed, a variety called the "sugar beet" is a major source of commercial sugar. Garden-variety beets are smaller and more tender. But they are still sweet, and a fine addition to carrot juice or any vegetable juice you care to name . . . and make. I greatly prefer beet-carrot juice to carrot-only juice . . . and I *like* carrot-only juice. Beets make the beverage better; they add flavor and nutrition that can't be *beet*. Sorry; too many years being brought up on pun-crazy Bullwinkle cartoons.

An interesting but weird side note: I notice less foam when I juice beets and carrots together. Just thought you'd like to know, as some people dislike foaming veggie juice. Another foam solution: drink it with a straw. One more juice excuse is ruined forever! Still not persuaded? Not hep to the jive? Well, then, maybe it's time to get out your grandparent's Cab Calloway records. (Many think he was first to use the word "groovy", and we're talking the 1930s.) At any rate, my name for beet-carrot juice is "Car-reet," as in Maestro Hi-De-Ho Calloway's famous exclamation, "Well, all *reet!*"

For further reading on beets, see our Recommended Reading section at the end of this book.

Cabbage

Cabbage is not particularly tasty, but it's particularly valuable when it comes to your health. High in both vitamins C and K, cabbage is also the source of Dr. Cheney's "vitamin U"—that vitamin found in those glasses of cabbage juice he gave—and healed with great success—patients with peptic ulcers. The food factors that the doctor collectively termed "vitamin U" are also found in the other cruciferous vegetables such as kale and broccoli. If you are feeling brave, you could run them through your juicer too. While cabbage may taste bad, it still heals gastrointestinal problems better than anything medically available. Juiced along with other veggies (and perhaps a fruit or two for some sweetness), cabbage can be worked into many recipes, whether you seek to treat a troubled tummy or not. Other than what we find in the coleslaw next to our Friday night fish fries, cabbage is not a hot menu item for many folks. Juicing is a great way to get more of this fantastically healthy veggie in our diets.

Carrots

I think we have said enough about carrots. Well, maybe not quite.

Besides drinking them on their own, carrots can be used as a foundation for many other veggie juice blends, and to disguise the taste of other nutritious but less-tasty vegetables like beets and zucchini (and cabbage!), as in "Car-reet," "Carrot-tini," and "Carrabage" juices. Adding a few apples or grapes to the mix is also a good way to get down the other less popular juices.

Celery

One of the most heavily pesticide-sprayed food products on the supermarket shelves, celery is not on our hit parade of veggies *unless you buy organic.* If you do, you will find that celery is a tasty addition to vegetable juices, as it provides natural sodium (salt). High in antioxidants, celery's good for the cells namely because its phenolic nutrients help prevent cellular damage.

Cucumbers

They are tasty, easy to grow, and cheap when in season. Go nuts: juice 'em all. If the cucumbers are organic, there's no need to peel them first. Most cukes are sprayed with pesticides, and then waxed so neither the rain nor you can wash it off. Solution? Peel them. Why drink them? Cucumbers are great for their antioxidant, anti-cancer, and anti-inflammatory benefits.

Lettuce and Other Leafy Greens

I grow leaf lettuce every year by the hundredweight and nobody wants it. Remember the story *Stone Soup,* where the villagers hid their food when the soldiers came to town? This is the opposite: some of my neighbors shy away (or outright flee) from me when I come around with bags of leaf lettuce. It's their loss. Fresh leaf lettuce, unlike supermarket iceberg, is a terrific food.

Try telling that to a teenager. I did. It sort of worked. When my son had a plateful of organic leaf lettuce put in front of him at dinnertime, he decided to run it through the juicer and drink it. You may prefer to eat it, but it can be juiced. Try it on St. Patrick's Day: the drinkin' o' the green. In fact, you can try it any day. Leaf lettuce is very easy to grow. Black-seeded Simpson is the cheapest, hardiest, lowest maintenance lettuce on the planet.

In addition to lettuce, *you can juice any green vegetable or green vegetable top that you could eat raw.* This means broccoli, cabbage,

HOT VEGGIE JUICE FOR COLD WEATHER USE

Feeling chilly? Live up north? Want something hot, and not that same-old liquid same old? Oddly enough, the human taste apparatus cannot easily tell the difference between physically hot and chemically hot. You can fake cooking without doing it. This can be good news for raw-veggie juice people. Radishes, or if you are truly a heat freak, hot peppers, added to your juice will heat it up without the stove. Pepper pointer: generally, the smaller the hot pepper, the hotter the hot pepper. A friend gave me (AWS) a peck (well, half a peck) of peppers. They were adorable, shiny, little red peppers, all nicely nestled together in the basket. Aw! They looked so cute and harmless, like little newborn vegetable kittens. Then I ate one, and all Hades broke loose. One dishful of ice cream later, I was able to reassess the occurrence. Moderation can be a wonderful thing if you have the sense to use it. So take a leaf from my life and go easy on the hot stuff until you know your tolerance point.

You have a time-hallowed alternative to cold juice, and that is hot soup. Yes, soup. On those winter days when I am feeling too darned cold to drink vegetable juice, I have a heated liquid decoction of the vegetables. A "decoction," to herbalists, is a boiled aqueous extract of the active ingredients from a plant root, stem, or leaf. Ladies and gentlemen, that's soup. As satisfying as hot tea, a large mug of hot vegetable soup warms your insides faster than watching you favorite sentimental movie. And it is nutritious. Although we constantly state and restate the benefits of raw, cooking has its place, and one of those places is certainly upstate New York when it snows. And snows. In Rochester, we expect a season total of about 7 feet of snow per year. Buffalo is no better, and Syracuse is worse: 10 feet is a "normal" winter. If that does not move you to soup, then try what I did: live in Vermont for a winter or two. When it snows up there, you can't get there from here. Hot soup is nearly as satisfying as a woodstove fire, and a lot less effort. More nutritious, too.

cucumbers (mentioned above), parsley, kale, Swiss chard, zucchini (mentioned below), young beet tops, carrot tops, or anything else your favorite rabbit eats. Tops are hard to juice. Add some water, or other high-moisture fruits or vegetables such as zucchini, tomatoes or apples. Or, entwine them around a carrot and put the parcel through as a unit.

Many and probably most juicing books go into the many virtues of green vegetable juices, and there is no need to reinvent the wheel here now. Green drinks are low in sugar but full of folate, vitamin A, vitamin C, and just about every other vitamin and mineral you can shake a rake at. However, green drinks look pretty unappetizing and tend to taste awful. Try adding some apples, pears, or even frozen fruit juice concentrate, for flavor. As for the color, close your eyes and think of England.

Tomatoes

Another goodie. For starters, tomatoes are high in lycopene, vitamin C, and beta-carotene. We know eating foods high in antioxidants is good to do. Let's get more of the good stuff and juice those 'matoes!

"Free Zucchini"

If you have not seen one of those signs on a roadside, you don't get out enough. The very huge, humpback-whale-sized zucchini that no one wants make very good juice. And lots of it. Not only that, the huge zucchini make *better* juice. Large, ripe squash are sweeter. Don't worry about all the seeds: most juice machines will remove them for you. In fact, I have found that the juicy squash, and the slight roughage of the seeds, cleans the inside of the juicer. Nice added benefit.

Growing zucchini is easy, and if you get any, you will get a lot. The price is right; the taste is tolerable. The health benefits are right on, too: zucchini is another good source of antioxidants. Juice zucchini with carrots to make my preferred way of disguising zucchini juice: Carrot-tini (trademark!). You'll even save more money, as you'll use fewer carrots per quart of product. I give my Carrot-tini to friends and family sometimes, not telling them what's in it. Always wait until the glass is empty before you tell them that they drank squash juice. Let the good times roll, and brace yourself for the verbal tirade (and be sure to duck the punches) that may ensue.

Orange-skinned kids. Lettuce-green drinks. Beet-red toilet water. Don't you just love this book?

JUICE FRESH PRODUCE

"Fresh" produce often isn't. Shipping, storage, and seasons are facts of agriculture. Fresh produce is best when truly cheap and truly fresh. Neither may be possible with today's high supermarket prices and long-term storage procedures. I think that turns a lot of people off to fresh fruits and vegetables. There is a fine alternative, though, and that is to grow your own. For just a few dollars worth of seeds, you can easily grow enough lettuce, squash, spinach, cucumbers, radishes, carrots, beets, and beans to last the entire summer at least. A 15-foot square garden can produce a tremendous amount of available-anytime fresh food. Even a window box or cold frame will grow quite a bit of lettuce and fresh salad greens through at least half of the year. Crop freezes, shortages, labor disputes, cash-crop market price fluctuations and all those price-hiker's excuses don't matter to the self-subsistent home gardener!

There are some fresh vegetables that you can buy nearly year-round at fairly low cost: carrots, onions, cabbage, and usually celery. These can be eaten raw or juiced, although why you'd want to juice an onion is beyond me. Squash, broccoli, leafy greens, and corn can be bought fresh in season at very low prices. You will no doubt be relieved that we quite agree that there is no need to juice corn. Corn is tasty eaten raw, right off the cob. You may be better off getting your fresh fruits at a roadside stand, farmer's market, or orchard. Prices are usually somewhat lower, and the fruit fresher when you buy directly from the producer.

Apples are a good example: I've seen apples for well over two dollars a pound in a supermarket, and there are very few apples in a pound.

At the same time of the year, at an orchard not far away, "utility" grade apples are fifteen dollars for a full bushel. A bushel would price out at only a fraction as much money per pound. *If you have any backyard at all, the trees to plant are fruit trees.* Dwarf varieties are easy to maintain and to pick, are ornamental, and provide a great low- or no-cost fruit source.

EASIEST, CHEAPEST CIDER PRESS ON THE PLANET: HOW TO MAKE YOUR OWN

The trick to making cider is to realize that whole apples cannot be pressed; you must grind them up first. I do this with a masticating ("chewing") type of juicer, which for this purpose I operate with all parts in place except for the juice strainer. This enables me to quickly run a large quantity of apples through it. I first cut the apples into quarters, both to check for critters and also so the apples will fit through the juicer's feed tube.

The coleslaw-consistency apple mash that the juicer produces is placed onto a good-sized cloth. I use old but scrupulously clean fabric salvaged from my worn-out rugby shirts, folded over into a nice, soggy, "appley" football shape and placed in my cider press.

Given the source of my straining cloth, by now you know full well that I was not about to spend any money on a cider press. My press cost me exactly nothing. I use a five-gallon, plastic, well-scrubbed, empty drywall compound bucket. I cut a piece of solid 1-by-12-inch pine plank scraps into two discs, which fit loosely inside the bucket. The bottom one has a couple of dozen quarter-inch holes drilled in it. The top disc is solid. The cloth-wrapped apple mash goes between the boards, and I put a couple of cement blocks on top for weight. Gravity does the rest.

To prevent such applied weight from jamming the lower wood disk into the bucket, I first place three stout plastic beverage tumblers, upside down, inside the bucket. The lower perforated wood disk sits on top of them. The cider collects in the chamber formed below.

Do not use plywood or composition wood for your pressing discs. In addition to containing some rather unpleasant chemicals in the glue used to make them, plywood, and chipboard products soak up liquid and will swell, distort, and quickly become unusable.

I've found that I can put about a half a bushel's worth of apples into this press at one time, if I prepare two large individual cloths of apple mash. I then get about a gallon and

Yes, Virginia, Fruits Are Good Too

If you make it (see inset below), fresh cider is a raw food, full of minerals and raw food enzymes. However, virtually all store-bought cider has been heat pasteurized. Like prepackaged carrot juice, it is still better than not drinking it at all. However, beware of supermarket "fresh-pressed" cider

a third of cider per pressing. That's better than two and a half gallons per bushel. (Times ten bushels: we are practically swimming in cider, and from only two apple trees.) You can let your pressing sit overnight, or you can perch yourself on top of those cement blocks, read your favorite natural health newsletter, and finish pressing in fifteen minutes. Kids love everything about making cider. If you are any kind of a Tom Sawyer at all, you can get them to literally line up to volunteer to be the ones sitting on top of the press.

When the pressing is complete, remove the cement-block weights carefully and set them aside. Then take the now-flattened (and much drier) apple parcels out of the press slowly; it is important that they do not open up, or your cider will instantaneously be transformed into extra-chunky applesauce. You see, as you lift them and lighten the load on the bottom wood disk, the disk will tend to float up on the inverted tumblers and sharply tilt to one side. Watch for it and you'll have no surprises.

Using a large funnel, pour your cider into storage jugs and refrigerate. Well, that's what I *officially* say you should do with it. You might, just possibly, er, ah, *forget* to refrigerate your cider for, say, a few days to a week. Should your memory happen to suddenly lapse to such an extent, join in the following refrain and have your designated driver handy:

Here's to thee, old apple tree,
Here's to thee, old apple tree!
Give us a crop of good apples ripe
Red and well rounded, the good juicy type!
Hats full, caps full,
Good bushel sacks full,
Our pockets, too:
Hurrah, wassail!

—OLD ENGLISH CAROL, AUTHOR UNKNOWN

VITAMIN C AND JUICING

Add vitamin C to juice as you make it: right into the receptacle to prevent oxidation.

Yes, add some vitamin C powder (available on the Internet and in health food stores), or vitamin C-rich cabbage or broccoli leaves, to your carrot juice and it will keep longer than it will otherwise. Vitamin C is a powerful and practical antioxidant. Prove it at home: cut an apple in two and rub some vitamin C powder on only one of the exposed halves. Wait an hour and compare the halves.

that reads in small print on the label, "preserved with one-tenth of 1 percent sorbic acid" or any other preservative. Real cider is just pressed apples, cloudy, dark, and perishable. Buy it fresh, read the label, and keep it cold. You can freeze cider if you are sure to leave one-fifth of the container unfilled to allow for freezing expansion (head room). I can easily drink three gallons of cider a week by myself. You might think that you'd get the "runs" if you did that . . . and you might at first. As your body gets healthier through a daily vegetable-rich diet, you'll find that it won't need to have the "runs" to clean itself out anymore, because it is already clean inside. Cider is sweet. Diluting half of it with water helps those desiring to keep their glycemic index (blood glucose) low.

It's incredible how much fruit you can get from a single fruit tree. One season, I picked about ten full bushels of apples from just two medium-sized apple trees. That sounds like an exaggeration, but it is, if anything, an underestimate. Being unsprayed, the apples are not two-dollar-a-pound showroom quality lookers, but, I have learned, they are eminently suitable for making cider.

"SO HOW MUCH OF THIS STUFF DO I HAVE TO DRINK?"

Drink as much juice as you wish. Remember that it is a food, not merely a beverage, and that you can have as much as you want. There is little fear of over doing it. It is, after all, hard to hurt yourself with vegetables. *Common sense caution:* use your noodle and work with your health practitioner, okay? If you are on medication or have any special health issues, discuss your juicing intentions with your doctor. Most physicians will be delighted that you are increasing your vegetable intake. If your doctor is not one of them, it is time to cut your losses and find one who is.

TRIMMING DOWN THE TIME IT TAKES TO JUICE

Unfortunately, juicing doesn't take a lot of time. If it did, it would be *so much easier* to avoid doing it. From organic-root-vegetable start to carroty-milkshake-goodness finish (including cleanup), the whole process is only about ten to fifteen minutes—really.

Nobody has a lot of time before work in the morning, but I (HSC) found this to be the optimal time to get my veggies. What a great way to start the day: knowing you have already loaded up on really good-for-you food.

Here are some tips for streamlining the process:

- Leave your juicer out on the counter, fully assembled, and near an outlet so you don't have to haul it around each time you use it. Yes, every visitor will ask, "What is that?" but it makes for a nice conversation starter.

- Keep your fridge stocked with organic produce. You won't feel the need to scrub everything for thirty minutes with gallons of soap and

---

FRIDGE FACTS

To keep your fresh produce fresh, refrigerate it. To keep it crisper, longer, try this:

- Store leafy greens in a medium-large crockery or glass bowl, topped with an upside-down dinner plate. This effortlessly maintains exactly the right humidity: not too wet, not too dry.

- Store carrots in their bag if the bag has some holes in it; if not, close the bag loosely to allow moderation in humidity.

- Green onions, green garlic (also called spring garlic or new garlic), celery, and similar veggies can be root-end down, in a non-tip cup or two of water.

water if it isn't laden with pesticides. Celery, spinach, lettuce, and peppers (mostly the above-ground veggies that are most exposed to topical chemical treatments) are great ones to buy organic, as they are very likely to contain the greatest amount of pesticides.

- Buy veggies that are "juicer-sized" when possible. If I spot a sack of jumbo carrots so wide I could use them for baseball bats, I skip that bag and find one with carrots that are much smaller in diameter. This way I don't need to split and trim and cut them down to size just so they fit into my juicer's neck. To save even more time, invert one or two small carrots nose to tail and juice at one time.

LEAVE IT TO CLEAVER

A good-quality, heavy, sharp meat cleaver is, oddly enough, the best tool to cut hard, tough, woody raw vegetables for juicing. Carrots tend to roll. Peeled beets tend to roll *and* be slippery. When you cut them, or anything, focus exclusively on what you are doing and use maximum caution. You do not want to have to buy a copy of our other book, *Lacerations: The Real Story*, now, do you? My (AWS) father always said that a dull knife will hurt you more than a sharp one. That is partly true, as a sharp knife goes straight into the target and is less likely to slide. However, sharp or dull, any knife can cut you and that's no joke.

I cut hard vegetables (such as beets) somewhat like I cut a pineapple or winter squash: I halve them first, so they will lie flat and pretty much stay put on the cutting board. I prefer large wood cutting boards. Yes, they will stain to the color of your vegetables. Think of it as wooden tie-dye. Far out!

- Don't bother removing end caps and stems on most items, unless they are surprisingly dirty, or starting to go moldy. For example, the ends of carrots or celery juice quite nicely, as long as they are as fresh as the produce they're attached to, so to speak. If the veggies are old and the ends and leaves have marinated in water in your fridge drawer, they can get slimy and rot. This is not very appetizing, and a quick trim would be advisable. However, if you have very fresh produce you aren't going to notice a difference in flavor if some tops, stems, and leaves go through the juicer too, and juicing vegetables whole saves oodles of prep time.

- Believe it or not, *not* hurrying will save you time. Press gently on the vegetable feeder-plunger and you'll get more juice and less heat. Do not shove the produce through. Let the weight of your hand and arm be sufficient. As your grandfather told you, let the machine do the work. Often, merely resting your hand on the plunger provides sufficient pressure to move the veggies through. Think of a juicer as a drill press with teeth. It will generate heat from friction. To reduce heat, add cold! Refrigerate not only the produce you are going to juice, but also the bowl or pitcher it is going into.

- Keep a compost pail (with filter) handy. Scraps sitting out in a bowl, or in your trash, become stinky rather quickly. The pail will prevent you from smelling the decomposing veggie byproducts, which in turn cuts down the number of times you need to dispose of the contents. Speaking of the contents, consider having a compost pile somewhere on your property (preferably out of the neighbor's view). Composting helps enrich the earth, it makes for great garden fertilizer and soil, and it also keeps organic waste from sitting in a landfill.

- You might think that juicing ahead and then storing it would really cut down on prep time. Indeed it would, except vegetable juice loses its nutritional value relatively quickly. To get the most out of your juice, drink it right after you make it. If you are going to put the money into buying the vegetables, buying the juicer, the work into raising a garden, and the time into making the juice, you may as well get the full benefit of the product.

Okay, so now you've got your juice, juicing byproducts, and a messy juicer. Let's trim some time off the rest of the process.

- Chug it down. There's no need to politely sip this beverage. You are in your home; nobody is looking. Go ahead and guzzle. Juice is the best for you when ingested immediately, so cut a few more minutes off your juicing routine by not wasting any time drinking it.

NOT NEARLY ORGANIC RADISHES

My (AWS) very first garden product was radishes. I was six years old. I planted them in a small strip of sandy dirt, on the side of my parents' house, in partial shade . . . and used the contents of our cat's litter box for fertilizer. My harvest was small. You may be relieved to know that I usually washed what radishes I harvested before consuming them. Francis Pottenger, Jr., M.D., was famous for his multi-generation nutritional studies on cats. He noted that cats fed conventional, cooked-food diets had manure (shall we say) that would not support plant life. I did not know that way back then, but now you and I both do. As comedian Benny Hill said, "Learning all the time!"

Vegetarian animal waste makes good fertilizer. It is vastly "cleaner" than carnivore droppings in both smell and bacteria types. I used to bring horse manure by the pickup-truckload from a nearby farm to work into the lousy soil surrounding our newly constructed tract home. In decades past I've also used cow manure. Chicken waste is even better, but stronger. Now I have a pet rabbit, and guess where *his* shavings and droppings go? Learning to garden organically, with mulch, compost, and no chemicals, is the right step in the right direction. See Appendix 2 on how to do it right.

- The moment you have finished making (and drinking!) your juice, just rinse the cleanable parts with water and set them in a dish-drainer rack until the next use. Soap will rarely be necessary as long as you don't mind the plastic parts of the juicer gradually becoming the same color as your favorite vegetables. A few swipes with a vegetable brush will help keep the juicer screen from clogging up from repeated use. Careful of dishwashers: don't use them for juicer parts. The plastic may warp or bend and misshape the pieces. Be fore-warned: All the vegetable bits are far harder to clean if you let the material sit and dry . . . then it *will* take forever to soak and clean them.

- Get another family member in on the action. Making juice for two is as easy as making it for one. Switch off the task, and you saved yourself some time every other day. Nothing makes juicing faster than getting someone else to do it for you.

MASTER'S CLASS IN JUICING:
Tips You Need to Know Before You Graduate

To get the most out of your vegetables and your machine in order to get the most into you, keep in mind the following. (Some of it you've heard before but it bears repeating.)

- Periodically clean the screen while doing a couple of quarts at a time.

- To get more juice out of the same quantity of vegetables, try putting them through your juicer more slowly. Gentle pressure works best; let the machine do the work. Taking your time juicing can yield as much as a third more juice. And, it will also reduce the heat from pressing vegetables too hard against the juicer's blade assembly. Reduced friction means cooler juice, which most experienced juicers consider to be better for you. Cooler juice also tastes better.

  Hint: A good way to check your juicing technique is to feel the discarded pulp. If it is wet, you are losing juice. If it is dry and puffy, you are extracting most of the liquid very well.

  Another hint: Clean the clogs as you go. Carrots and other veggies can be very fibrous at certain times of the year. This is all the more reason to slow the juicing process down a tad. But if you are really going at it, stop juicing every five pounds or so, unplug the juicer, and (carefully) rinse off the blade assembly under running cold tap water.

- Keep up with juicer maintenance. That sharp blade may dull over time, but it will probably take years and years. If you do happen to notice decreased juicer performance, hop online or call up the manufacturer and order a new blade. Sharp juicer blades juice better as do sharp knives slice better.

- For those who can afford it, there are some very fine, albeit very expensive, juicers that press the vegetables rather than spin a blade against them. While there is little question in my mind that juicer-presses are ideal, a lot of people simply cannot manage their high cost. I'd rather you juice cheap than not juice at all. Better juicers tend to yield more juice. As a ballpark estimate, to get about six glasses (1.5 quarts) you need to juice about five pounds of carrots. That sounds like a whole lot of carrots. But it's not really: there are only about two dozen large carrots in a five-pound bag.

- Add vitamin C powder to the juice as you make it. It keeps the juice from (darkening) oxidizing until you drink it.

- Drink first; then rinse all liquid-contact, non-electrical juicer parts immediately.

- Don't like foam? Drink your juice through a straw.

- Try to always buy organic. Not only is organic produce pesticide-free, not only does it encourage more organic farming, not only is it better for you and for the world—*it freakin' tastes better!* What's that? Well, sorry! Just because it's a master's class doesn't mean it has to be dignified.

"WHAT ABOUT WHEN YOU ARE TRAVELING?"

If you are on a car trip, take your juicer. It is smaller and quieter than most dogs. I have never seen a motel sign that said "No Juicing."

If you are travelling by air, ask for tomato juice as your in-flight beverage. Drink veggie juice before you go and after you land. Drink it while you are at your "final destination." I mean, you *are* going to deplane, aren't you? You can find a grocery store almost anywhere. Many sell canned, boxed, or frozen vegetable juice. All these are far, far better than nothing. V-8 has been widely available for decades. It is canned mixed vegetable juice. If you are buying canned, try to get the reduced salt product. Beware of "juice drinks," "splashes," "cocktails," "drinks," or anything that is not 100 percent pure vegetable juice. Otherwise, you will likely be paying for substantial fractions of sugar and water. Canned juice tastes better cold. Very cold.

LESSONS FROM DOWN UNDER
AND UP NORTH

Exercise is king, nutrition is queen.
—JACK LALANNE (1914–2011)

When I (AWS) studied in Australia, I went for a pleasantly romantic walk with a coed late one evening, and looked up. The night sky was "wrong." I mean, no Big Dipper? What kind of a hemisphere was this, anyway? My fascinating discovery did not take away from the joy of the moment, and is hardly reason to not date science majors. But these may be: I learned on an arid uphill-both-ways daytime hike (with a different coed) that you should not sit on bulldog ants. And, from that same young lady, that then (1973) kangaroos were still made into meat pies, and the country's immigration policy was openly racist. Much has changed in forty years, and good on you, Australia.

A mate of mine at Australian National University was a strict vegetarian. I thought he was nuts. But I also noticed he was invariably healthy, and one of the calmest people I'd ever met. As for me, I was still eating meat pies and sausage rolls, their shady origins notwithstanding. My diet was pretty awful back then. And, while theoretically in the very prime of youth, my own health was no better than marginal. Did I immediately change my ways? Of course not. I suffered along, like so many folks still do, in the sure-and-certain knowledge that vegetarians were extremists and that health is to be obtained by prescription.

Two years later found me in Vermont. Talk about a far cry from Down Under: I can tell you that Vermont autumns can be powerfully cold. I wore two shirts, a sweater and a coat, when my friend Doug was serenely walking around the village half naked. No, he was not an exhibitionist, just a hippie. He really looked the part, man. Long, long reddish-blond hair, a beard (which he actually kept well trimmed) and, of course, sandals (when he wasn't barefoot, which was usually). Pretty much all he wore were cut-off jeans and, when the snow got too deep, boots, and perhaps a light jacket. That's it.

In a close-knit mountain village, where everyone spent half their time within arm's length of a woodstove and the other half of their time bringing wood in to it, this guy stood out just a tad. As for clothes, well, he must have saved a pile at Sears.

I had to ask him why he dressed so lightly all the time. "I'm just doing as the Indians did. I've found that I get acclimated to cold if I don't worry about it so much." While I suspect that Native Americans probably like warmth as much as the next person, the real message was that what Doug did seemed to work for him. He was one of the healthiest looking people I've ever met, and while not a muscular guy by any means, he had dawn-to-dusk endurance. Doug and his wife had a little boy. I closely observed this beautifully healthy, mellow yet active vegetarian toddler on many occasions. Like father, like son: he did not wear a shirt, either.

I have, over time, tried dressing more simply and dressing light, à la Doug. It works. I was once introduced at a health food store as the "famous Dr. Saul." The person replied, "He doesn't look famous to me." If you dress Doug-style, you will probably get this a lot.

But doing so may have a weight-loss benefit. Burning calories is not just done by exercising. Your body temperature is close to 100 degrees Fahrenheit. That means even on a warm, nearly 80-degree day, the atmosphere is cooler than you are by 20 degrees. Hmm. On a 40-degree day, the outdoor temperature is nearly 60 degrees colder than you are. You are burning food-fuel calories just to keep warm. There has to be a weight-loss program in here somewhere. Being outside is probably associated with more activity. I submit that it can also help you keep trim just by getting used to, and even enjoying, being in the cold. Cold also drives you into activity. When I walk, or work in the garden, the chill of the underdressed is indeed tangible stimulation to keep moving.

Popular fears of "catching a chill" are based more on myth than medicine. Polar Bear Club members should, by rights, be more scarce than honest politicians if it were otherwise. As kids, we went off to camp in upstate New York for several weeks each summer. We swam in cow ponds, wallowed in puddles, and fell into creeks. We were always getting soaked. Dry sneakers were the sign of a wimp. We played dodge ball in the rain and had swimming lessons, outdoors, in the rain, no matter what the temperature. On overnights, we slept in leaky canvas tents and froze by morning. No, the Rochester YMCA was not trying to kill us; this was just "roughing it" and it did us nothing but good. And our parents, who willingly paid hard-earned cash for us to have the experience, were not conspiring to do us any harm, either. Probably. It all built character.

People strain at a gnat and swallow a camel. Nature is not your foe. Get off your gluteus maximus and go outdoors. Shake that body! Move it! Feed it a plant-based diet! Make your own heat, and watch your mood soar and your doctor bills dive.

WHAT DID PEOPLE DO BEFORE JUICERS?

Perhaps they pressed produce between heavy rocks? Certainly the wine press and cider press hint at some juicing along history's way. Primarily, though, they chewed their food. Some people have taken this to the extreme of very nearly juicing with their choppers . . . literally.

Fletcherism

"Eat your juices and drink your food" would most succinctly summarize the philosophy of Horace Fletcher (1849–1919). Without ever mentioning the name Fletcher as far as I recall, my mother adhered to his precepts. Mom tried, utterly in vain, to get my brothers and me to "chew our food thirty-two times before swallowing." No chance of that; at our dinner table, my hungry and older brothers followed their own Darwinian precept: survival of the fastest. No grass grew under their forks, let me tell you. After downing the lion's share of available victuals, one brother raced out to go and play basketball; the other vanished to some other part of the house to play stringed instruments.

Don't eat "until you are good and hungry" was another Fletcher maxim that I first heard, over half a century ago, from my mother. She was unknowingly quoting him. My guess is that my great-grandmother had something to do with this, but it is far too late for me to verify. What we do know is that he had a point there. Only eating when truly hungry is truly good advice for the majority of our overweight modern population. Indeed, Fletcher himself was overweight and suffered from indigestion. This led him in 1895 to experiment and then passionately espouse thorough mastication of all foods. While not a physician, he can not be dismissed as uneducated. Fletcher was a graduate of Dartmouth, had a master's degree, and was a fellow of the American Association for the Advancement of Science.

Don't gobble your food. Fletcherize, or chew very slowly while you eat. Talk on pleasant topics. Don't be in a hurry. Take time to masticate and cultivate a cheerful appetite while you eat. So will the demon indigestion be encompassed round about and his slaughter complete.
—JOHN D. ROCKEFELLER

Fletcher "taught that all food must be deliberately masticated and not swallowed until it turned to liquid. Fletcher believed that prolonged chewing precluded overeating, led to better systemic and dental health, helped to reduce food intake, and consequently, conserved money."[6]

He travelled, wrote, and lectured extensively. And he was very successful: Fletcher became a millionaire at the time when there were not many of them, and millions were very big numbers. Alternately called the Path to Dietetic Righteousness, or the "Chew-chew" cult, depending on whom you asked, the approach certainly did no one any harm, and may have done John D. Rockefeller some good. He Fletcherized, and lived to age ninety-seven. Yes, I know that correlation does not mean causation, thank you. Let's keep that scientific thought in mind when we consider this next sentence: Fletcher died in Copenhagen in 1919, at age sixty-nine, of what was considered to be bronchitis. We may bear in mind that the post-World War I years (1918–1919) saw the most deadly flu pandemic in history. It was especially rough going in Europe. Linus Pauling's advice about taking lots of vitamin C would fit well.

If you would like to read more, in Fletcher's own words, see the following publication: Fletcher, H. *Fletcherism: What Is It*. London: Ewart, Seymour & Co., 1923. Reprinted by the Lee Foundation for Nutritional Research, Milwaukee, 1960. A free full text download is available at http://www.soilandhealth.org.

Nightingale Was a Naturopath

It's true. Florence Nightingale, the mother of modern nursing, was a health nut. So was American Red Cross foundress Clara Barton. All the very best nurses (and doctors), past and present, are health nuts.

As I always say: If you're not a health nut, then what kind of a nut are you, anyway?

And what exactly is a health nut? Someone who eats right, lives right, and feels right. A health nut is upbeat; eating right will do that for you. A health nut is active and productive. Interviewing very elderly people reveals that they have one thing in common: they all have something that they absolutely, positively *must* do tomorrow. I believe that health is also about fearlessly doing the right thing. Reforming medical care, for example.

Hygienic nurses Florence Nightingale and Clara Barton raised a real ruckus in the medical profession. It was, after all, bad enough that they were women! Their century was an era virtually devoid of female physicians. If you could ask your ancestors if they had a woman for a family doctor, you'd get precious few "yes" answers.

Furthermore, the woman doctors that did practice were usually graduates of homeopathic and naturopathic schools. Today, we tend to be quite unaware of this.

That may be because we were never told. "Pharmaphilic" physicians like to parade Elizabeth Blackwell's 1849 graduation from Geneva Medical College as heralding the first female doctor of "modern medicine." The wonderful educational and charitable work of Dr. Blackwell will stand for all time. But politically correct (pharmaceutically correct?) history has slipped quietly, and I think deliberately, by the real story: nineteenth-century women of medicine had their roots and their practices in herbal, hygienic, and nutritional therapy.

An interesting paper entitled "Naturopathy, Nightingale, and Nature Cure: A Convergence of Interests" by P. McCabe and published in *Complementary Therapies in Nursing and Midwifery* in 2000 has helped to fill in the facts.[7] Says the author: "An examination of her writings supports the hypothesis that nature cure was a significant influence on Nightingale's understanding of health and healing."

Here's a Nightingale favorite: "The very first requirement in a hospital is that it should do the sick no harm." In her ninety-year life (1820–1910), she and Clara Barton (1821–1912) would say it often. Note both of their lengthy life spans.

We need these ladies again, now. Hospital stays are more dangerous than ever, killing some 300 people every day. That's a jumbo-jet full, dead, every day.

Clearly, we need to apply natural, nutritional commonsense and gumption today. That means organically grown whole foods and fresh vegetable juices for every hospital patient. Don't tell me this is "too expensive." What's one single day in the hospital cost? Hundreds (even thousands) of dollars? And for this, they can't tack on an extra twenty bucks for organic food, fresh vegetable juice, and some supplements? Doing so would automatically minimize the need and consumption of medicines, and consequently reduce unnecessary deaths. Of course, it would also pretty much empty out the hospitals. Well, there's your explanation for why it's *not* being done.

Our hospitals are themselves sick. Hospitals are still nearly as deadly as the unsanitary hospitals Florence Nightingale and Clara Barton knew so well. Take action now. Be a health nut. Be an activist. Walk the walk, and talk the talk, and juice.

6

GERIATRIC JUICING

An elderly woman went to a new doctor. Right from the start,
he said to her, "You realize, of course, that I cannot make
you younger." She replied, "I do not want you to make
me younger, doctor. I want you to make me older."

—OLD STAND-UP JOKE THAT EVERY COMIC
STOLE FROM EVERY OTHER COMIC

Fresh out of college, with Emerson and Thoreau in mind, I (AWS) lived up in the hills of Vermont. My elderly friend Maurice LaSalle, an octogenarian of French-Canadian extraction, and I were talking one day. I said to him, very facetiously, "Maurice, I'm getting old."

He thought about that for a spell, giving it far more consideration than it was worth. Presently the old gentleman answered, with a slight smile: "Then keep right on!"

I took that to mean that if you keep right on getting older, you are still here. I mean, consider the alternative! Remember the teaching of one of history's great yogis (Yogi Berra): "It ain't over until it's over."

Should you be afraid that it might be too late for you, remember this: if you are alive, you have time since 98 percent of the atoms in your body are replaced every year. Just think: 98 percent of you is *brand new* in only twelve months. And every one of those atoms can only come from what you breathe, drink, and eat.

If you are sick and tired of being sick and tired; if your get up and go has got up and gone; well, here's some help: start vegetable juicing today.

YOUR TURN IS COMING

What, today? As in "now"? Yes, now. Because there are only three possibilities: (1) you are old already; (2) you will be old; or (3) you will never make it to be old. If you do not relish choice three, listen up and plug in. The elderly are the number one users of a developed country's medical and hospital services. Perhaps this is why most of my experience with older people is with the very ill. From the elderly who are just now learning natural healing methods for the first time, I frequently hear this:

"If only I'd done this thirty years ago!"

It has been said that the number one regret of an aging person generally is not about something they'd done badly, but rather about something they had never tried to do at all. Sometimes, that is something as basic as eating right and exercising. There is nothing to lose, and a lot to gain, by giving your health priority in your life right now, regardless of your age.

As for my outlook on aging, I shall never join the American Association of Retired Persons (AARP). Unless, of course, they change the name of their magazine back to *Modern Maturity*. And if you like musical satire, be sure to listen to the Tom Paxton song of the same name, released in 1996. AARP dropped that title in 2003. Maybe it was a coincidence. Personally, I like over-the-top kitschy titles. If I cannot have dozens of issues of *Modern Maturity* scattered throughout my house to annoy my children, then no deal.

Eighty-Nine and No Meds

When it comes to juicing, doctors generally do not know much about it, and generally they don't want to know. That's why it is so much fun to quote Nancy Watson Dean, an elderly lady who had an organic garden in the middle of the city of Rochester, ate a natural diet, juiced, and took vitamins. In her eighties, she was in the hospital for a hip replacement. Nurses came to her room from other floors to meet the woman who was on zero meds. She was outspoken.

Nancy Watson Dean, age eighty-nine:

> Lots of money can be made from drugs and knives. What would the medical industry do if everybody lived as I do? I finally said to my doctor: "What's the point of me coming for appointments with you when you can never find anything wrong? Let's stop wasting our time!" He agreed, so I just call him for things like injuries.
>
> For my first sixty years I followed the medical route, having allergies, colds, sometimes the flu, some joint replacements, and more. I thought that was what life was like. Then I started following a natural lifestyle. Soon I noticed I no longer had my allergies or flu or even sniffles. I have no ailments, no prescriptions, and am actively pursuing my art, with commissions and profits, though I am now eighty-nine. I wrote this in a letter to a doctor at the Mayo Clinic. He never replied (*Doctor Yourself Newsletter,* March 5, 2005).

Age ninety:

> Focusing on so-called vitamin overload risks is lot of prattle. What is risky is not taking vitamins. I take lots of supplements every day, and absolutely no prescriptions at all. I have no ailments, and I will be ninety-one next month (*Orthomolecular Medicine News Service,* May 22, 2006).

Age ninety-two:

> This is the approach that is big in Europe, but doctors here hate it and don't allow it to be taught in medical schools or made available to their patients. It produces a person with no ailments, allergies, or prescriptions. I have been on it for years. I love not having to waste time being sick! (Personal correspondence, 2008)

Nancy Watson Dean still took no medications, dying peacefully of natural causes at age ninety-three. At home.

JUICING AND HOSPITALS

"Jim! You can't leave him in the hands of twentieth-century medicine!" said Dr. McCoy in *Star Trek IV*. Some things are known to just not mix. There's oil and water, and then there's fresh vegetable juice and hospitals.

A hospital, by definition, is a collection of the sick, the injured, the infirmed, and the stressed. All these situations call for larger than the normal quantities of nutrients. When is the last time you saw a hospital or nursing home routinely give even a daily multivitamin, let alone fresh-juiced produce? Another silly little plastic cup of processed, cooked-and-filtered-to-oblivion apple juice will not do it. Neither will another few ounces of orange juice concentrate. We are talking pints— pints of fresh liquid veggies here. Those who disagree can take their food groups and put them where the FDA doesn't shine.

Prepare to stand firm on what is most important, and negotiate the rest. Here are our suggestions:

• If you want to juice while hospitalized, bring the juicer with you (and preferably a person to operate it and guard it and you). A written statement from your doctor that you will be doing so may save a lot of fuss. I'm not exaggerating: hospital staff often tell patients they may not take anything that the hospital didn't authorize them to take. You can hardly count on them to provide fresh juice. So it is a bit like a movie theater telling you that you can't bring in your own popcorn, but they won't sell you any, either. Staying alive is vastly more important to an enjoyable hospital stay than popcorn is to a movie.

• If you want to bring premade juice into the hospital, prepare it as fresh as you can, right before you visit. Put the juice into a prechilled Thermos or similar insulated container, and fill it literally to the brim. This reduces air inside, and thereby reduces oxygen, and consequently reduces oxidation. Also, dust the top of the juice with vitamin C powder. Vitamin C is a potent antioxidant, and it will help keep the juice tasty and nutritious longer. Or even better, stir in the vitamin C powder before you fill the container. Does it really matter? Remember that you can test it and see for yourself. Try one batch with vitamin C and one batch without. Note the more intense color in the vitamin C-treated juice. Without it, the juice will, in a matter of speaking, brown, like lettuce overlong in the fridge or an apple cut and abandoned.

- If you are given a plausible medical reason why you should not drink fresh juices, be bold and ask for written scientific references. Look up each surgical procedure or medicine you are offered. If a vegetable can be eaten raw, then it can be juiced. Is there *really* a problem with a vegetable? Sometimes. Warfarin (Coumadin) dosages may have to be tricked-out if you consume a lot of vitamin-K-rich leafy greens. Grapefruit interferes with some drugs. So it is best to check. Complete information on drugs is contained in the *Physician's Desk Reference (PDR)*, which can be found in any hospital pharmacy, library, or doctor's lounge. Your public library will probably even look it up for you if you telephone them from your room. It is also online. Have your personal family bodyguard bring their laptop along with the vegetables.

  The *PDR* lists all prescription medications (there is another book for nonprescription medicines) with all their side effects, contraindications, and any nutrient/drug interactions. It is quite rare for vegetables to interfere with a prescription drug. Any such caution is in the *PDR* in writing. The same information is on drug package inserts. Do not assume that you doctor or nurse has memorized the nutrient/drug connections of the thousands of drugs in the *PDR*. Also, do not piously accept the dumbed-down "About Your Medicine" handouts that you may be given with a medication. Go to the *PDR* and read the unexpurgated version.

  Surgical information may be obtained from sources other than your surgeon. Try an Internet search, or the public or hospital library for non-technical books like *Good Operations, Bad Operations* by Charles Inlander (Penguin, 1993). To know every aspect about any surgery proposed for your disease, two standard reference works are *Greenfield's Surgery: Scientific Principles & Practice*, 5th ed., by Michael W. Mulholland, et al. (Lippincott Williams & Wilkins, 2010) and *Schwartz's Principles of Surgery*, 9th ed., by F. Charles Brunicardi, et al. (McGraw Hill, 2009).

By the way, any doctor or nurse who makes fun of you for being thorough probably should be more thorough themselves. Don't stand for harassment, especially when you are in the right. Tell a supervisor. If that doesn't work, write to the hospital's board of trustees, the newspaper, the Better Business Bureau, your congressperson, the local newspaper. See why you need that laptop? If you have no laptop, borrow one. There must be a teenager somewhere in your extended family.

START EARLY

While I (HSC) was in the hospital maternity ward, recovering from childbirth, I drank a lot of vegetable juice. The lactation specialist was all smiles when she saw the big containers of carrot juice. She said it was so good to see that because it would provide such great benefits for both the baby and me. My daughter got lots of carrot juice in her first year. She's now in her second year, and we're not going to let up now.

Unacceptable Reasons for Stopping Juicing

If by juicing you are looking for a standing ovation from your local hospital, HMO, or medical society, you are going to have to look mighty hard. Once you become a juicing health nut, you can expect to be dissuaded by pretty much every medical professional you are obligated to talk to about it. Here's a sampling of what you may hear:

- "Juicing will interfere with your tests." Just have the words "drinks vegetable juice" added on to any paperwork. If necessary (and it is very unlikely), an interpretation can readily be made. If there is a specific and essential test or procedure that clearly requires suspension of vegetables, you can stop the day before and resume immediately after it is over. This way you only lose a day.

- "Juicing will be dangerous after surgery." Since all nutrition textbooks indicate a substantially increased need for nutrients and fluids after surgery, this objection is illogical.

- "Vegetable juices are unnecessary if you eat right." I say, long hospital stays are unnecessary if they *fed* you right. Since they don't, fresh juices are the simple answer. If you find a hospital that feeds you a vegetarian, three-quarters raw food diet (blended or juiced for some patients, as needed), then I will lighten up. Until then, hospital food will continue to deserve its almost pathogenic reputation, and supplemental juicing is completely justified.

- "We have our rules." Baloney. It may be their building, but it is your body. Accept nothing without an explanation that is satisfactory to you. If the nurse or doctor or aide or clerk or orderly or anyone else "says so," ask for a supervisor. If the supervisor "says so," ask to see the hospital administrator. If she or he is "too busy" for such contact, leave. There are other hospitals. If this sounds like shopping for a new car, well, it very nearly is. Only this is more important.

  Remember, all bureaucracies are most sensitive at the top. Schoolchildren (unfortunately) know that the principal is more likely to be understanding than the teacher they just talked back to. The board of education will be even more attentive. Do not argue with a nurse, doctor, or hospital staff member. Demand to meet with top authority if there is any unresolved problem. No hospital executive wants bad publicity. Perhaps, after a tirade like this, you expect me to grab my broomstick and wail, "I'm melting!" I have no apology to make for asserting your right to assert your rights.

Hospitals provide essential services and save lives. They will save even more when they fully utilize the one piece of technical apparatus that they do not have that will do you the most good of all: a juicer. As Yogi Berra said, "You don't have it, that's why you need it."

Hospitalization Juicing Checklist

Know before you go. It is immeasurably easier to get what you want if you contract for it beforehand. Prenuptial agreements, new car deals, roofing and siding estimates, and hospital care need to be negotiated in advance. When the tow truck comes, it is too late to complain about who's driving—same with an ambulance, or a hasty hospital admission. You have to preplan, and here's how:

1. **Get a letter.** Yes, a "note from the doctor" still carries clout. Have your general practitioner, today if possible, sign a letter stating that he backs your request for an in-room juicer, all the vegetables that you desire, and a lot of Dixie cups should you (or your designated loved one) require hospitalization. Have copies made and keep them handy. Update the letter annually. You now have your GP's permission. Good start, but not enough.

2. **Get some more letters.** Obtain a similar letter from every specialist that you have used, are using, or may use in the foreseeable future. This sounds cumbersome, but is no more unmanageable than most people's grocery lists. Keep it in perspective: this is just as important as wearing a medical alert bracelet or keeping a fresh battery in Grandpa's pacemaker.

3. **Make some calls.** Telephone a representative or two from every hospital within 100 miles of your home. Find out which wants your business the most. When you find a "live" person on the phone, write down his or her name and title, and follow up with a letter.

4. **Write for your rights.** In your letter, ask for the hospital's assent to have a juicer on hand should you or your designated family member(s) come in to that hospital. You must get this in writing. Now, do *not* say, "I want that in writing," because people do not like that. But if you *write to* them by U.S. postal snail mail, they will naturally write back to you. Bingo. Helpful hint: In this case, do *not* correspond by email; you want a real signature on hospital letterhead. (And no, don't ask for that either! It will happen automatically if you write first.)

Possible replies:

- "No." You might be wondering, What if they write back, "No, we won't." Hold on to that letter. You can make a real stink with it should you need to play hardball in court, and I do *not* mean a handball court. But threatening malpractice is the mating call of the loser. Avoid the very mention of "attorney" and you will probably get further, quicker, and certainly cheaper.

These following are much more likely, however.

- No reply whatsoever. Sometimes, they simply will not write back. Okay, so ask yourself this: What if your credit card company didn't respond to your letters? So would you entrust your life to a hospital that refuses to even answer their mail? Make a point to go someplace else. If you live in a rural community or a smaller city, you might be thinking that you do not have a choice of hospitals. This may be the case for the first twenty-four hours in an unexpected circumstance, but people can be moved. That's what modern transportation is for. Famous hospitals get people from all over. How many people do you know that live within walking distance of Sloan-Kettering, Roswell, or the Mayo Clinic?

- Useless reply. What is more likely is that the hospital's representative will send you a garbage answer, with a response so non-committal as to be unusable. This may mean that you wrote the wrong person, or wrote the wrong letter. Try this: have your doctor write the letter. By that I mean the doctor's letterhead and signature, your composition. Go ahead; you can give a professional a rough draft of what you want said. The doctor has staff that can easily rewrite it on office stationery and the doctor can sign it. It saves time. Helpful hint: be sure your (doctor's) letter clearly *requests a reply.*

- String-along reply. It is also quite possible that the hospital will ask for more information. This could be a genuine interest, but it is more likely a stall. If they ask you to telephone and discuss it, they want to get it off the record and avoid a paper trail. Don't fall for that one. If you think there was some serious fiddling whilst Rome burned, you should see what medical bureaucrats can do. To cut through the treacle, you need to understand the nature of the beast. The first rule of lion taming is, you have to know more than the lions. Therefore . . .

5. **Know the law.** Many states have enacted legislation that makes it possible for a physician to provide any natural therapy that a patient requests without fear of losing his or her license. If your state has such a law, it will make it somewhat easier to get a doctor to even specifically prescribe juices.

6. **Know the power structure.** Find out who is in charge. I have heard doctors say that they'd be happy to comply, but the hospital will not let them. Then, when asked, I have heard the hospital say that they allow what you are requesting, but the doctors won't do them. To avoid an endless catch-22 situation, you have to know the ropes and where everybody stands.

   - On the doctor side: Which physician (as opposed to witch doctor) is in charge? It could be the attending surgeon; it could be your general practitioner; it could be the chief resident. One thing is for sure: someone has the power to prescribe. Go to the person that can do you the most good (or harm) and start your negotiations there. If you can persuade the king, the castle is yours.

   - On the hospital side: Which of the administrators has the clout? Talk to their secretaries (they are the people who really run things anyway) and you will find out. It could be that the most influential person for you may be the hospital's patient rights advocate or VP for customer service. It might even be the public relations director. Who knows? You sure don't, so remove the veil of anonymity and find out.

   - On the patient side: The patient, if conscious, has all the power because it is his or her body. If a patient insists loud and long enough, he or she can get almost anything. Since patients tend to be sick, and therefore easily slip into becoming non-combatants, a family member has to get in there and pitch for them. Let's return to the mention I made earlier urging you to make sure you have your own personal bodyguard. This is not hyperbole. A highly experienced nurse told me that she would never leave a family member in a hospital without a twenty-four-hour-a-day guard in the form of a friend or family member or other advocate. That is sound advice from a lady who's seen it.

Next to the patient, the most powerful family member is the spouse. After that, it would be children. You do not have to have power of attorney to have power, but it helps. If the patient is unable to speak, act, or think, it may be essential. Do not wait until the patient is incapacitated to plan this. Your family needs to come together (difficult though this may be) and present a preplanned, unified front to the medical and administrative people. You may think I am overstating the case, but *I have seen hospitalized patients die simply because they did not receive water or food.* Juice is both. If the patient can eat or drink, they can have juice.

7. **Know the facts about vegetable nutrition.** For this, there is absolutely no alternative to reading up on the subject. At the conclusion of this book we have a Recommended Reading list with a few comments about each entry.

   I juice a lot, and quite frankly, there are many days when I do not want to. I am, however, extremely interested in saving life, including my own. The reading I referenced above may make all the difference in your case.

8. **Know how to settle controversy and avoid the run-around.** Doctors and hospitals are quick to offer rather bogus reasons why they would deny or interfere with your decision to drink juices. Each of these arguments is a lot of bull, and easily refuted. (There are more non-institutional excuses in the next chapter titled, oddly enough, Juicing Excuses.)

THEIR ARGUMENT: We do not have any juicers.

YOUR RESPONSE: So get one. I hear the big-box discount stores are open 24/7.

THEIR ARGUMENT: We have never done this before.

YOUR RESPONSE: Then this is a wonderful opportunity to learn. I've never lost a (insert family member's position here) before.

THEIR ARGUMENT: The patient is too ill.

YOUR RESPONSE: That's why we want juices. They are nutrient-rich, easy to absorb, and require no chewing. If the patient is able to eat or drink, they can have juice.

THEIR ARGUMENT: We might get into trouble if we do this.

YOUR RESPONSE: You will avoid trouble, you will avoid bad publicity, and you will make me happy if you do this.

THEIR ARGUMENT: There is no scientific evidence that this is safe, effective, appropriate for this case, blah, blah, blah . . .

YOUR RESPONSE: Read this. (This short phrase is to be spoken as you produce a large stack of juicing books. No need to put this book on the top unless you really want to.) We also want you to read the books in our Recommended Reading section and the articles in our Reference section.

THEIR ARGUMENT: But we do not have time to read all that material.

YOUR RESPONSE: That's okay. I already have, and it's my body (or my father's, or my mother's). Here's what to do: *Plug in the juicer. Juice these vegetables. Offer them to the patient. Throw away the cup. Repeat every snack time and every mealtime, and do not stop it without my written authorization.*

Confrontational? Admittedly, yes. But I have seen too many people die too soon. I have no nice way to phrase this: I'll be damned if that is ever going to happen again if I can prevent it. Don't let it happen to your family.

7

JUICING EXCUSES

The secret of life is honesty and fair dealing.
If you can fake that, you've got it made.
—GROUCHO MARX (1890–1977)

We are very good at finding reasons *not* to do something. As far as I'm (HSC) concerned, it's one of the easiest things to do. It is in our nature. It is far simpler to not act than to bring something to action, especially when it involves our health. Action takes energy. Action requires motivation. To stick with something we have to be determined. We can't allow our excuses get in the way of doing what we know to be right.

When we introduce new routines into our lives, there are always barriers to overcome. Something is bound to get in the way if you let it. There are probably thousands of reasons why we could put off juicing vegetables—and most of us do. Don't you miss out on an opportunity to change your life for the better. Let's take a moment to address some of the more common "stoppers" that keep us from juicing, so we will be more likely to start.

Here they are, in no particular order.

JUICE EXCUSE #8   I Don't Know What to Juice

Anything. Almost. (Try to avoid your fingers.) If you can eat it raw, then you can probably juice it. Of course you'll want to focus on veggies, especially ones you like, but don't be afraid to try new combinations or toss some fruit in there to sweeten things up a bit.

If you still don't know where to start, begin with carrots. As you become a more confident juicer, add other ingredients to that "CJ" base. Carrots juice easily, they are sweet and tasty, there's little prep work needed, and they are amazingly good for you. If this book seems CJ-centric, it's because it is. Carrot juice is a really great foundation for many other veggie juice blends, especially those that the authors like!

My (HSC) favorite juice blend:

Carrots (5 or 6 large)

Cabbage (1/4 medium-large head)

Beet (2 small or 1 medium)

Cilantro (small handful)

Yield: About 1 pint

My (AWS) favorite juice blend:

Carrots (about 12 large)

Zucchini (2 medium or 1 large)

Cucumber (1 medium)

Apples (1 or 2)

Yield: About 3 pints

Want more ideas? Go online or grab a juicing recipe book. Someone out there has already done the work for you. They have come up with all sorts of yummy combinations that will help you avoid any experiments going awry, and subsequently down the drain. Please check out the juicing recipe books listed in our Recommended Reading section at the end of this book.

JUICE EXCUSE #705   Finger Juice

All juicers require common sense caution. Juicers are power tools and should be used with respect. Follow all manufacturer's instructions. Your children may help you in age appropriate ways, but do not let them juice alone. Supervise your kids. The first thing to tell them is what you just read above. I (AWS) told my kids, "Be careful, or you'll have finger juice." They understood instantly and there was never a mishap. Most juicers are designed with great care to make finger juicing all but impossible, but experienced parents know that nothing is really impossible when it comes to children. Humorist Sam Levinson said that when he was a boy, his mother used say, "Go see what your brother is doing and tell him to stop it." When my son was three, we told him not to put a bean in his nose. Do I have to finish the tale?

JUICE EXCUSE #41   I've Heard Carrot Juice Has Too Much Sugar

"Glycemic index" is the amount of sugar in a food. Some root vegetables are fairly sweet, notably beets and carrots, which are so emphasized in this book. There is method to our madness. Folks, the problem with the American diet and American obesity is *not* that we are eating too many beets and carrots. *This* I (HSC) know for sure. A far easier way of overdosing on sugar would be to gobble down a package of gumdrops. It is healthy to eat, and to drink, your vegetables—yes, even carrots. The nutritional benefits of carrots far outweigh the natural fructose present in each root. The same goes for beets.

If you are diabetic or have other known blood-sugar issues, you should be cautious. Work with your physician. While so doing, bear in mind that consuming more vegetables of any kind, in any form, virtually guarantees a lower glycemic index than eating carbohydrates or fruits, juiced or otherwise. We are not against complex carbs and we are not against fruits. We are *for* eating and drinking more vegetables more often. Sweetish vegetables taste good and are therefore more likely to be juiced and regularly consumed by real people. If you are a purist, go for green drinks. Juice cabbage, kale, leaf lettuce, wheatgrass, and other greens. They are all low in sugar. They are also low on most people's hit parade of taste bud treats.

JUICE EXCUSE #16   I Turned Orange—Not Cool

Okay, okay. I suppose that is a little weird. It's also completely harmless. Hypercarotenosis occurs when you eat a large quantity of beta-carotene rich foods like sweet potatoes, carrots, pumpkin—the obvious culprits since they wear that distinct color—and your skin actually turns orange-yellow. Reminiscent of a bad fake-tan, it too will fade if you juice less.

If you keep juicing a lot, you are likely to be perpetually carrot-tanned. A good bout of influenza or pneumonia will get rid of the excess carotene. But you don't want that, and if you juice, you are less likely to get sick. Still, excess carotene is like a savings account with a passbook that every passerby can see. Personally, I care not. We're here; we're orange; get used to it!

JUICE EXCUSE #5   It Doesn't Taste Good

The better it tastes, the more likely you are to drink it. It's pretty hard to get excited about juice (or get your kids interested) if it tastes awful. While some folks may say to steer away from sweeter additions like apples or carrots, I'll argue that adding flavor this way is the right idea *because it gets the juice down*. For example, if salad dressing makes a huge salad more appetizing, add some. A little fat and salt goes a long way when you are eating like an herbivore. If you can stomach a salad dry, have at it. But for the rest of us who need to "dress-up" our veggies before we take them out, herbs, citrus, apples, and beets can brighten up a juice drink that would otherwise not appeal to you.

JUICE EXCUSE #27   I Don't Know Which Juicer to Buy

The one that you will use. Think of all the expensive exercise equipment folks purchase . . . and barely touch. A person can buy the fanciest, most technologically advanced machines on the market, but these feats of modern engineering don't do their owners a lick of good unless the purchasers actually *use* them.

The same is true for your juicer. If you are a hesitant consumer, maybe try a simple juicer first and see if you use it enough to warrant an upgrade. You can always buy a better one later, and give your "starter" juicer to a friend. For example, a casual baker might need only a hand mixer to blend an occasional bowl of flour, sugar, and eggs. A more serious chef may need to get that heavy-duty standing mixer that will last years and years and handle every job, big or small, that it's given.

JUICE EXCUSE #73   Juicers Are Too Expensive

Some cost a pile; you're right. But others are very inexpensive, with a price tag that is comparable to a month of cable TV. If you are just starting out, maybe you aren't ready to make a huge investment in a juicer. Then don't! Start with something relatively inexpensive, keeping in mind the old adage: "You get what you pay for." Machines that cost more may indeed be much better quality. They may be more durable and do a better job extracting the most juice out of each vegetable. Over time, a more efficient juicer will pay for itself because it is less wasteful of the produce you buy.

JUICE EXCUSE #2   It Takes Too Long

This *would* be a good excuse except it isn't true. At our house, juicing takes about ten to fifteen minutes from start to finish, including cleanup. Check out tips for "Trimming Down the Time It Takes to Juice" in Chapter 5 for more helpful hints.

JUICE EXCUSE #99   Vegetables Are Too Expensive—Especially that Organic Stuff

Relatively speaking, vegetables aren't that expensive: it's prepared foods that are. Don't want to buy organic? Then buy some soap—one that lacks a strong "flavor" or scent. Wash your produce with soap and water to remove as much pesticide as possible. Rinse thoroughly to avoid a sudsy aftertaste. Non-organic produce is cheaper, and if that makes you and your wallet happy, and gets you to juice more often, that's good!

JUICE EXCUSE #12   It's Gonna Kill Me

Alas. We are the sad victims of our five o'clock news programs. We have reason to fear, that vegetables are going to do us in. How often have little green onions, spinach leaves, and lettuce heads been in the news media marked as "Dangerous!" because they have been exposed to *Escherichia coli* (*E-coli*)?

Perhaps we need to take a moment to reflect.

Nasty little microbes show up on our produce not because vegetables are fundamentally hazardous, but because they have been handled improperly.

The solution? Stop eating vegetables. Just kidding.

What you should do is wash your produce. Yes, you can use soap. A drop or two of suds goes a long way in helping remove anything you don't want present on your produce so you can receive the health benefits of continuing to eat raw foods. There's no need to go cold turkey and ban the broccoli.

Vegetables are good for you, and often much more so than other foods. For some more fun, check out Appendix 3: "Another *Reader's Digest* Absurdity: Red Meat Is Bad—No, Wait—*Good* for You!" and make up your own mind about red meat. (And no, we're not a vegetarian, but there is much value to be found in veggies.)

COLI CALMING

E. coli fears on spinach and other veggies? It is not the plant's fault. *E. coli* is the bowel bacteria. Wash your hands; wash your veggies. And do not overthink this. If you have ever had a swim in a cloudy green-water lake, creek, or pond, you've been exposed to *E. coli*. As kids, we learned to swim in a cow pond and spent more time in pre-treatment-plant cityside lakes than you'd ever believe. And yet, here we are. Why? Nature has given you an immune system. Plus, your body's digestive tract contains good bacteria that keep harmful bacteria from taking over. Eating yogurt, a high-fiber diet, and taking vitamin C also help.

Cooking food does kill bacteria. But we cannot live in a heat-sterilized bubble. Raw foods are healthy, and juiced raw foods healthier still. (Remember why? Not denatured by heat, greater intake, better absorption.)

JUICE EXCUSE #451 **Beets Contain Oxalic Acid, and Oxalic Acid Causes Kidney Stones**

Right on both counts . . . but there is more to it than that. We discuss this issue in Appendix 4, "How to Prevent Oxalate Kidney Stones."

JUICE EXCUSE #35   A Glass of Juice Doesn't Stick with Me

Well, what else are you eating? You shouldn't be attempting to survive on juice alone, unless you are temporarily detoxing or juice fasting. For us casual juicers, we also should be seeking out healthy sources of protein and good fats which aren't found in bags of endive or green beans. Juice doesn't have to take the place of a meal, and for many of us it shouldn't. It should be *part* of our healthy diet and arguably, a big part. If you are in a hurry, a hard-boiled egg, a spoonful of natural peanut butter, some butter on toast, or a handful of nuts can be a quick way to get some fat and protein in a hurry. Otherwise, juice and then eat a normal meal too.

JUICE EXCUSE #42   I Don't Think It's Worth the Effort

Don't think vegetable juicing is going to make much of a difference in your life? Don't think it's worth it? I challenge you to give it a try for two weeks and then make up your mind. When I was younger, my dad always said to me to read the first chapter of a book or watch just the first ten minutes of a movie; if I didn't like what I was reading or watching after that preview, then I could move onto something else. Before you make any decisions about juicing, give it the ol' college try first. When you see how great you look and feel, you won't need much convincing!

JUICE EXCUSE #321   I'm Just Too Busy

Too busy to juice? I say you are too busy *not* to juice! Juicing is fast and efficient. It's quicker to drink your veggies than to chew them. The busier you are, the more stress you are under, and the more your body needs, *craves*, great nutrition. Why not get all those vegetables your body needs anyway, the easy way!

JUICE EXCUSE #64   My Spouse Doesn't Support My Decision to Juice

No matter what your new healthy life change might be, it is always tricky when you lack support. If your partner "sabotages" your efforts, consciously or not, it is very difficult to stay on course.

Are you being picked on because you are drinking vegetable juice? "Ew! What *is* that? Why do you drink that stuff?"

(Remind you of the middle school lunch table, anyone? Anyone?) Or, is there any other spousal scenario that makes it difficult to follow through on your goal? For example, let's say a husband (or wife or partner) decides to work out every day. He is looking great and his health is benefiting, too. A nonsupportive spouse may make it difficult for him to find time to work out; she may make him feel guilty about it for one reason or another because she feels down about her own appearance. A fit spouse makes it all the more apparent that the other is not. The same can be true when it comes to what we eat.

It can be difficult to make changes to your diet. It's even harder if your family isn't on board with your decision to do so. Sometimes folks like company when they make suboptimal health choices. Your spouse may count on you for this kind of company. Nothing eases a guilty conscience quite like getting someone else to make a bad decision with you.

Another scenario: it is extremely hard to say no to junk food when it stares you right in the face, so one of the best ways to avoid sweets is to simply not have them available. Changing what is brought home from the grocery store means not everyone in the household will be happy about it. "But we've *always* bought these. We like them!" These are difficult battles to win.

It's a whole lot easier to do something good and healthy in your life if you have support. If there are people that get in the way of you doing what is good and healthy for *you*, you have a more difficult task than those who don't, that is true. We guess this is when you find out how determined you really are.

AFTERWORD

Now that it's finished, just remember . . . that it's not.
—RINGO STARR

When a good friend of mine (AWS) had serious, relentlessly painful gastrointestinal problems that doctors and medicines could not relieve, he drank juiced broccoli leaves for a week. He hated it. And all his gastrointestinal problems went away. He now appreciates juicing a lot more. Neither this nor most other examples of juice-use show a love of liquefied vegetables. But there is no faster, easier, more effective way to get down quantities of veggies than juicing. As authors, we have the easy job: all we have to do is write. You have to go and do all the work. Well, not exactly. We are subject to the very same rules of nature that you are. We are all in this together.

INFAMOUS JUICING LINES FROM FAMOUS LITERATURE

The quality of vegetables is not strained . . .

Friends, Romans, countrymen: lend me your produce.

Quoth the raven, "Power on!"

Thank you for having successfully withstood our a-peeling (or appalling) sense of humor. If you have read this far, you should already have a carrot juice moustache. Or be about to go and get one, right now!

APPENDIX 1

———

AN INTERVIEW
WITH ANDREW W. SAUL

by Nancy Desjardins (www.HealthLady.com)
March 18, 2010 (abridged)

If you'd prefer to listen to this interview unedited, go to http:// health-lady.com/audio/InterviewWithDrAndrewSaul.mp3.

Nancy Desjardins: Dr. Saul, what first attracted you to natural healing and inspired you to write *Doctor Yourself, Fire Your Doctor!* and especially, *I Have Cancer: What Should I Do?*

Andrew W. Saul: Probably the thing that made the biggest impact on me was when my first child was born. I was the old age of twenty-two. They put the baby in my care and said, "Here, Dad." Looking at that child and then watching the hospital mishandle him for the next day or so convinced me that I had to do something. In fact, I took my wife and son out of the hospital after just a day—which at the time was short—in a raging blizzard against the nurses' and the doctors' orders because they were making my child sick, and my wife, too.

I knew something was wrong. I could see that. They were feverish. They were fretting. They weren't eating. They were getting ill. I took them home, and then I was faced with the question, "Now what?" You can't just say no to medical care. You have to say yes to an alternative. The alternative has to be at least as effective, and certainly had better be a lot safer.

My reading and my experience over the last thirty-four years has taught me that orthomolecular medicine, or nutritional medicine, is the safest and most effective way to prevent and treat illness.

ND: For our listeners, I'm so big into juicing. This is something that I've been promoting for several years for everyone. Again, if you just joined in our call tonight, we have Dr. Andrew Saul. This is interesting. Like with juicing, it's such a part of my daily routine because I've been juicing for many years now first thing in the morning. This is my breakfast. I juice my vegetables. It's green, leafy vegetables, and I add some carrots, apple, ginger, kale, and Swiss chard, and I feel amazing. It's great. Also, this is going to be a protocol that I'll be using in my seven-day detox program. I was very happy to see, Dr. Saul, that you have an article on juicing as well.

AWS: There are several of them, absolutely. I'm a big juicing fan. At www.DoctorYourself.com, do a search for "Juicing," and there are several articles. It tells you what to juice and how to juice it. It sets out a way that you can encourage your family to do juicing. Fresh, raw vegetables are good for you.

When you juice them, you have to understand what you're actually doing. When you juice vegetables, you're only doing two things: first of all, you're breaking down all the cell walls and releasing all the nutrients, and you're doing that without cooking. Juicing gets you better absorption. You get better absorption because it's been liquefied. The second thing you get with juicing is you get quantity. When you juice, you can drink a quart and a half of juice down in no time.

Because juicing gives you more absorption, you tend to have higher quantity. Better absorption and higher quantity means better results, whether it's vitamin C or carrot juice. Don't let anybody dissuade you from juicing. Vegetable juicing is a tremendous help. In fact, the Gerson cancer therapy is based on juicing.

Dr. Max Gerson was a German physician who fled Nazi Germany right before the Holocaust. Gerson came over to the United States, fortunately, and began practicing in the Long Island area of New York. Dr. Gerson was known as a migraine doctor. He had terrible migraines himself. He tried everything. He tried all kinds of drugs and other therapies. Nothing helped. Finally, he decided to try nutrition. And, by golly, when he started eating organic, fresh, unprocessed, natural, good foods from the garden, he found his migraines were relieved a great deal. And, when he started putting these vegetables through a juicer and increasing absorption and quantity, he got rid of his migraines.

People started coming to see Dr. Gerson to get rid of their migraines, and he became rather popular. Gerson noticed that his patients were not only getting over their migraines, but they were getting over other illnesses as well, including tuberculosis and several other very serious illnesses that he writes about in his books.

There were people who came to Dr. Gerson and said, "Dr. Gerson, would you please treat my sister? She has cancer." Gerson said, "No, I will not. I am not going to get in trouble with the authorities. I'm not going to be known as one of those quacks who treats cancer. I'm sorry. I can't do that." They pleaded with him, and Gerson decided to take the chance. He started having cancer patients eat a whole-, organic-, unprocessed-foods diet with no salt, virtually no sugar, reduced protein, and up to twelve 8-ounce glasses of vegetable juice a day.

What he found was that the juices detoxified the body and helped the liver to recover. He believed the liver was the key organ to fight cancer in the body. Gerson was getting a very good cure rate. In fact, using juices and nutrients, Gerson's cure rate for terminal cancer was around 50 percent, which is extremely high. For malignant melanoma, his cure rate was spectacular.

Dr. Gerson went before the U.S. Congress in 1946. They were talking about fighting cancer and what should be employed. Gerson said, "In addition to the other things, you want to consider nutrition." Gerson, unfortunately, was disregarded. Surgery, chemotherapy, and radiation were accepted and, more importantly, funded, whereas nutrition was put on the back burner. We've been suffering ever since.

ND: Going back to how many ounces, it's 96 ounces per day. That might sound crazy to drink 96 ounces of vegetable juice, but it's really doable.

AWS: I've done it!

ND: Absolutely. I've done it too, and I know for many of my clients and participants, that's what they do when they do a juice fast or a juice cleanse, especially if you're going to do a seven-day or fourteen-day juice cleanse. By the second day you just feel amazing. On the third day, you have a lot of energy. Actually, with Dr. Gerson, it's Dr. Gerson's daughter, Charlotte, who's one of the experts.

AWS: Charlotte is a very healthy eighty-eight [2010].

ND: That's right. Our next question is from Joyce in Nashville. "Are all cancers the same, and can they be treated the same? For example, blood cancers, lymphomas, and tumor-growing cancers."

AWS: It's a good question, and the answer is no and yes. Are they all the same? No, otherwise oncologists would always do the same thing for everybody and textbooks would only be short pamphlets. Are they all the same? The answer is yes in that, according to Dr. Max Gerson, they're all a product of a toxic body that needs more nutrition. We have undernourished, overfed bodies. In some cases, there's exposure to chemicals.

In any event, the Gerson approach, and in many ways mine, would be to say that we're not really treating cancer. We're treating a person who has cancer. We're treating the person, and when we treat the person, we want to basically do two things. We want to build up the person's immune system so his or her own body can fight the cancer. Unfortunately, modern medicine doesn't do that. Modern medicine tends to go in and remove the cancer surgically, which isn't a bad idea; it's just incomplete. They also zap it with radiation. That's not a bad idea, but it's just incomplete. They could also give chemo drugs that are poisonous to cancer. That's not a bad idea, but it has terrible side effects, and it's only 3 percent effective.[1]

What modern medicine doesn't do is use aggressive, high-dose nutritional therapy. That's what we need to do. All hospitals need to do this right away, and I'm here to tell you they're not going to. You have to fight for this. Fortunately, you can because if you really push hard, you can get your hospital to allow you to juice. It's still a really scary situation. The good news is that there's more than you know. There are more choices. It isn't just cancer therapy with radiation, chemo, or sur-gery. You have more options. You can use nutrition. I think, at least in my thirty-four years, every cancer patient I've worked with has had increased quality of life and increased length of life.

ND: Absolutely. Our next question is from Bridget: "My husband has prostate cancer. He had his prostate out three years ago. Two years ago, he had thirty-three radiation treatments, and last year he started on hormone shots. He has hot and cold flashes. I'm looking for a natural cure without the ugly side effect."

AWS: There are many things you can do. One thing that sometimes isn't mentioned is lycopene. Lycopene is the red stuff in tomatoes. It's basi-cally what makes tomatoes or watermelon red. Lycopene is a very strong antioxidant. It's even stronger than carotene. There have been a number of studies in Italy, which isn't terribly surprising, where they found that men who eat ten or twelve fresh tomatoes a day had a much lower chance of getting prostate cancer.

There have been other similar studies done. In Japan, for instance, they found that eating sea vegetables, seaweeds, fish, and tofu, avoiding red meat, and having more of a low-fat, healthy diet reduces risk of prostate cancer. The Japanese have much lower rates of prostate cancer than we do. If the Italians and the Japanese can do it, so can we. I think you need to understand that nutrition is probably the part of the ther-apy that has not been looked into by your oncology team. It's up to you to read about it. There's no shortage of information. You just have to get out there and take a look. There's a lot of good news. There are no easy answers, but there are answers, I think.

ND: That's right. This is our last question. It's from Dennis. I had to share this one. "My wife passed away four years ago after three years and eight months of battling inflammatory breast cancer. She went through sixteen different protocols of chemo, thirty-eight radiation treatments, and four surgeries. Why didn't any of [the] many clinics and doctors say anything about diet and nutrition?" You answered that question.

AWS: That's very powerful. I want to remind everyone listening that the wife of one of my coauthors died of cancer. Another one of my coauthors had a couple of grandparents die of cancer. I had two cousins, both younger than me, and one a lot younger, die of cancer. We have all felt the pain of this disease. That's why we wrote the book *I Have Cancer: What Should I Do?*

For you and I and everyone listening, we have to get out there and change this. We can't wait anymore. People are suffering, and it's time to put an end to it. Nutrition does help. Is it the total, 100 percent answer? No. Is it a big part of the solution? I think it is. You have to use enough, and you have to be sure it happens. You can't assume the hospital is going to provide good, healthy food. They won't. The hospital is not going to provide juices. The hospital is not going to provide them unless you make it happen.

I have a nephew who's fourteen. Do you know how hard it is to get a fourteen-year-old to eat right? He saw *Food Matters,* and this was a kid who just lived on junk food. After seeing the film, my brother (his father) told me that he heard him out in the kitchen after the movie saying, "You are what you eat. You are what you eat." He started eating good food and lots of salads. I think it's wonderful.

Linus Pauling, the only person in history who has won two unshared Nobel Prizes, is the scientist who named orthomolecular medicine back in 1968. Linus Pauling said, "Don't let anyone make up your mind for you. Check and see for yourself."

APPENDIX 2

———

BEGINNING YOUR ORGANIC FOOD GARDEN

by Norm Lee

To forget how to dig the earth and tend the soil
is to forget ourselves.
—MAHATMA GANDHI (1869–1948)

(AWS) Back in the 1980s, every summer we loaded the family into our truck with the camping cap on the back. We were once again on our way down to Naples, New York, for the Home-steader's Good Life Get-Together. These annual events were organized by Norm Lee, a dedicated activist, homesteader, and organic gardener. If you want to save bucks and eat better, here is a good summary of what Norm would recommend you start with. I have known the author for decades now, and he is still right on. Grab a shovel and join in. (Used with the kind permission of the author.)

ONE: THE BASICS

Why Garden?

As the gardener tends his plot and seasons pass, the more benefits he likely realizes. He or she may begin with the single aim of reducing food bills, then find the flavors are far superior to the supermarket's. With the extra vitamins and regular mild exercise comes a gradual improvement in general health and vigor. News of a trucker's strike brings no stress. The confidence and security derived from independence from expensive stale produce and killing frosts in far-off agri-biz fields cannot be estimated in dollar value.

As produce ripens so grows the pleasure in sharing lore with other gardeners, as gardeners have practiced since man evolved from hunter and gatherer to gardener and home builder. Now the garden begins to be recognized as a quiet and patient teacher waiting for the gardener to open to its subtle and profound lessons. One may begin to experience spiritual joys as the garden, once a mere work place for "digging in the dirt," evolves into a refuge, a retreat for mindful meditation.

Why Organic?

The home gardener chooses to grow organically so his plants can feed on nutrient-rich, natural soil instead of artificial fertilizers, and he declines to play the fool by spraying poison on his food.

Site: The plants require a reasonably level site with minimum six hours' sunshine, access to water, and soil conditions that allow for deep-dug compost beds. Choose a spot that is protected from strong winds, away from trees and large sun- and water-hogging bushes. Southeast of the house is best, due south next best, east is third best; forget west and north. In southern and southwest areas of the United States be sure to provide 50 percent or so shade protection during summer months.

Soil: Gardening is like good parenting: you think first always in terms of meeting the needs of the garden. You take care of the soil, the soil provides for the plants, the plants produce food for you. So the three most important things in gardening are: soil, soil, and soil.

In most areas there are three types: clay, sand, and humus. It is good to have a mixture favoring humus, but in any case your soil will improve with compost. Be an extremist here; composting cannot be overdone. No need for home gardeners to test for pH. As a general rule, whatever the problem or deficiency of your soil, lots of compost will fix it.

Compost: The organic gardener is not troubled with poor soil, because wherever he is, he makes his own. I've raised gardens in Vermont, three sites in New York, and three sites in Arizona. In a Mexican fishing village I developed a deep-compost food garden on the salty, sandy shore of the Sea of Cortez. All successfully grew abundant food. There is no soil that cannot be improved by composting.

There are many compost "recipes," but providing your garden with sufficient compost is not mysterious, complicated, nor work-intensive.

Layer a few inches of each: topsoil (humus), greens (grass clippings, raw vegetable kitchen scraps, leaves), manure (horse, cow, or chicken— never dog or cat). No meat. Keep the pile moist but not wet, and aerate it by mixing (turning) it every few days. After a few weeks (composting is not an exact science) it will be ready to spade into your garden soil, or fill up garden beds, and/or use as mulch.

> *Behold this compost! Behold it well . . . !*
> *It grows such sweet things out of such corruptions.*
> —WALT WHITMAN

Mulch: Mulch is compost-type material used to cover the soil's surface after the plants have started. Other than compost, mulch is by far the best friend and work saver a gardener ever had, far better than any $2,000 rototiller. Apply two or so inches of grass clippings, peat moss, leaves, chipped Xmas trees, bark, pine needles, the list is nearly endless. People even use newspapers, old carpets and flagstone, but these do not feed nutrients to the soil as do the above.

TWO: THE METHODS

Why not combine the best gardening methods known today? You want practices that (1) produce the most abundant crops in the least space; (2) provide the most vitamins, flavor, and economy; (3) require the least work, water, and tools, (4) most effectively deter harmful insects, plant diseases, and weeds.

Organic methods deliver [the] healthiest produce, most economically.

The composted soil produces [the] largest crops, and makes for the strongest plants—which insects like to avoid.

Raised beds, once built, are work-savers in many ways: more efficient use of compost and mulch, smaller garden to fence and shade, and more production per plant (because the soil is not compacted by treading between rows).

Intensive planting combined with deep mulch-raised beds multiply food production per square foot many times over. The "shade mulch" keeps down weeds, keeps soil moist, and saves water.

Companion planting has been proven to discourage predatory insects; basil among the tomatoes, for example. In fact, scattered plantings of French marigolds, onions, radishes and any mint herb will do much to discourage the bad bugs, but keep good ones like lady bugs and mantis.

Successive plantings can easily double your food production by extending the growing season alone. Beginning with starting seed flats of tomato and cabbage family in late winter, you can raise a spring garden, a summer garden, and a fall garden.

Year 'round gardening. In the late '70s, early '80s, I pioneered a method of producing vegetables all winter long in the outside garden in northern climes, eliminating the need for greenhouse, root cellar, freezing, drying or canning. Our New Year's Day vegetarian meal consisted of twenty vegetables bursting with flavor, fresh-picked from raised beds under a blanket of dry hay, sheet plastic, and a foot of snow.

Natural foods will be the medicine of the future.
—THOMAS A. EDISON

THREE: PLANNING

Your Paper Garden

Stage (1) of gardening is doing your reading; Stage (2) is creating the plan. These can be as enjoyable as the stages following: (3) digging in the dirt, and (4) plucking the harvest. The most common things to not do:

- Don't use chemical fertilizers or pesticides
- Don't plan a large garden
- Don't plant rows instead of beds
- Don't fail to use compost
- Don't plant too much seed too thickly
- Don't buy many "work-saving" tools
- Don't plant seed too deep
- Don't fail to apply mulch

How to Avoid Work

The wise (and lazy) gardener plans a small garden, loads raised beds with deep compost, and plants intensively. This reduces losses from pests, diseases, and drought. The raised-bed intensive planting uses the compost, water, and mulch most efficiently, reduces the stooping and bending, and virtually eliminates weeds. There is no plowing, tilling, hoeing, cultivating, weeding, spraying, dusting, etc.

You can quickly spend $2,000 on tools, sold to you on the claim that they "save work." When you calculate the hours of work required for the money to pay for them, those expensive tillers and weeders, and sprayers are not so cheap. You need only four tools: a shovel, a rake, a trowel, and a four-tine fork. In hotter climes, a hose for irrigation.

Tools that *make* work: rototiller, hoe, cultivator, plow, harrow, seeder, chemical sprayer, and sprinkler.

What to Plant

1. Easiest to grow: radish; leaf lettuce; spinach; tomato; onion sets; sweet corn; summer squash; beet green; bush bean; turnip; pea

2. Quickest to harvest: six weeks—radish; turnip; leaf lettuce; spinach; bean; beet greens; summer squash, green onion from sets

3. Most popular vegetable in home gardens: tomato, leaf lettuce, onion, cucumber, beans, radish, green pepper, carrot, peas, beet, spinach, corn, summer squash, cabbage

4. Most nutritious vegetables: (in order of food value, fresh and raw); broccoli, spinach, Brussels sprouts, lima beans, peas, asparagus, artichokes, cauliflower, sweet potato, carrot

5. Short season crops: bush bean, beet green, cauliflower, cabbage, carrot, lettuce, radish, pea, early corn, Chinese cabbage

6. Flats to set out a month before average last frost in spring: cabbage; broccoli; cauliflower; onion; lettuce; Swiss chard

7. Flats to set out two weeks after average last frost date: tomato; summer squash; green pepper; cucumber; eggplant, cantaloupe

When to Plant Seeds

1. Plant on the last frost date: beans, corn, cucumber, pepper, cantaloupe, pumpkin, summer squash, winter squash, watermelon

2. Plant at mid-summer: Chinese cabbage, parsnip, pea, turnip

Space to Allow

Minimum space requirements per plant:

2 inches: peas, carrot, green onion, beet green

4 inches: bean, dry onion, parsnip, spinach, turnip

6 inches: leaf lettuce, celery, cucumber

9 inches: Swiss chard, potato, spinach

12 inches: Chinese cabbage, head lettuce, potato, sum squash, tomato

Normally potatoes, sweet corn, squashes and melons are grown in patches, not raised beds.

> *"When the world wearies, and society ceases to satisfy,*
> *there is always the garden."*
> —MINNIE AUMONIER

ANOTHER *READER'S DIGEST* ABSURDITY: RED MEAT IS BAD— NO, WAIT—GOOD FOR YOU!

by Helen Saul Case
for Orthomolecular Medicine News Service

Browsing through the July 2012 issue of *Reader's Digest,* it's not those witty "Laughter Is the Best Medicine" sections that are making me chuckle. It's the ridiculous, contradictory health advice that the magazine gives to the reader.

Let's start with what makes sense. In the article "Is Meat Good or Bad for You?"[1] the author explains that red meat might be killing us. He references a Harvard study[2] that tracked over 121,000 adults for up to twenty-eight years and shares with us that *"people who ate three ounces of red meat every day were about 13 percent more likely to die—often from heart disease or cancer—before the study ended than people who didn't eat meat."*[3] And, folks who eat processed meat fared worse. They increased their risk of early death by 20 percent. This sounds like pretty important information, not to be taken lightly. He writes, "It's no wonder that many experts recommend reducing or eliminating red meat from your diet." That's certainly true.

Alas, the author's common sense ends there. As my grandmother said, "Common sense isn't common." Well, Grandma is right again.

The author mentions in his rebuttal that regular eaters of lean beef get more protein, zinc, potassium, and B vitamins. Ah yes, protein. Good thing we have red meat! I mean, you can't find adequate amounts of protein in *anything* else but red meat. Except for beans, of course.

Oh, and cheese. And it's also in tofu, nuts, lentils, eggs, yogurt, milk, seafood, and more. Still, how do those vegetarians survive? Apparently they do, if the Harvard study is to be believed, and in greater numbers than the meat-eaters.

Okay, vitamins and minerals sure are important. You can't get them anywhere but in a steak. Yeah, right.

With all that evidence the author just provided, we still want to know the final verdict: is red meat good or bad? Apparently, "You can still fit a daily serving of red meat into a healthy diet."[4]

Really? A "daily serving" is considered to be about three ounces. Awesome! I get to eat three ounces of red meat a day!

Wait, didn't the Harvard study *just say* that three ounces of red meat a day was killing people? Did the author read his own article? Qualifying the eating of red meat by using the phrase "as part of a healthy diet" makes about as much sense as the huge bowl of sugar-laden breakfast cereal pictured on the front of the cereal box that boasts being "part of a complete breakfast." But this is only when presented next to a pile of whole-wheat toast, fresh fruit, orange juice, and a pound of spinach. Okay, I made up the spinach part.

So, red meat is bad for us. But, according to the article that said so, we're supposed to go ahead and eat it anyway.

Isn't that what the reader of the *Digest* takes from the article? Must be. In the oxymoron box (or maybe just the "moron" box) entitled "How Healthy Carnivores Eat," it recommends the "perfect" portion of meat is about the size of a deck of playing cards. Perfect for what? A coronary? Goodness knows, when many people eat red meat, the serving is larger than any "deck of cards" outside of a novelty shop. Nor will this advice likely prevent Americans from consuming their 100 pounds or more of red meat a year, an amount way out of proportion to our intake of fruits and vegetables.[5] Oh, but if red meat is a part of a *healthy* diet, we'll be A-okay, says *Reader's Digest*.

Uh huh. Because that's your average American: fit and healthy. Eating lots of vegetables every day to deliberately offset that chunk of red flesh. Oh, please. Only about 30 percent of us get either two servings of fruit or three servings of vegetables,[6] and only 11 percent of Americans are meeting U.S. Department of Agriculture (USDA) guidelines for both.[7] Surveys have found that there are a whopping 20 percent of folks out there that eat absolutely no veggies *at all*.[8]

Is it really so daring to recommend we skip red meat altogether? Would the *Digest* lose subscribers? Would the *Digest* lose advertisers? Well, they must be losing somebody, because the advice in the article encourages continuing to consume red meat and risk death and disease.

Folks, we don't need to chow down on cow to obtain our daily dose of zinc and B vitamins. Vegetables have plenty.[9] And though the carnivore in us may be quick to disagree, plenty of widely available plant-based protein-packed foods can be placed in the shopping bag. Healthy sources of potassium are easy to find. Virtually all fruits and vegetables are an excellent source of potassium.[10] A vegetarian diet, selected with care, provides generous amounts of protein and all the other essential nutrients necessary for excellent health.

So, let's see . . . eat red meat and risk death. Or, skip the meat, actually try to eat the healthy diet we *should* be eating anyway, packed with vegetables. And, while we are at it, take vitamins and eat fresh fruit. I think that's doable.

Do yourself a favor and don't "digest" *Reader's Digest* ridiculousness. Toss it in the trash bin, and you'll actually be a whole lot healthier for it.

APPENDIX 4

PREVENTING OXALATE
KIDNEY STONES

Your body, and the bodies of animals in general, manufacture an organic substance called oxalic acid ($C_2H_2O_4$). You also consume it in your food. Some vegetables, such as rhubarb, okra, spinach, Swiss chard, sweet potatoes, and beets, contain a considerable amount of oxalate (the form of oxalic acid in food). A variety of other vegetables and fruits contain at least some oxalate. Oxalic acid can combine with calcium in the urine to produce calcium oxalate, a compound that can crystallize and clump together to form a calcium oxalate kidney stone. We include the following adaptation of material originally appearing in the peer-reviewed *Orthomolecular Medicine News Service,* which may help clarify this issue . . . and very possibly your urine as well. (Adapted with permission, February 12, 2013; for the full text, see http://ortho-molecular.org/resources/omns/v09n05.shtml.)

Vitamin C

Gorillas are vegetarian and eat a lot of plant foods. This means they eat, and make, quite a lot of oxalate. A gorilla also gets about 4,000 milligrams (mg) of vitamin C a day in its natural diet. The U.S. RDA (recommended dietary allowance) for vitamin C for humans is only 90 mg a day. The gorillas are unlikely to all be wrong. However, if your doctor advises that you are especially prone to forming oxalate stones, read the suggestions below before abandoning the benefits of beets, vegetables in general, and vitamin C in particular.

The oxalate/vitamin C issue appears contradictory. Oxalate is in calcium oxalate kidney stones (the most common type). Oxalate stones are common in humans but not common in gorillas. Ascorbate (the active ion in vitamin C) may slightly increase the body's production of oxalate. Yet, in practice, vitamin C does not increase oxalate stone formation. Emanuel Cheraskin, M.D., D.M.D., (1916–2001), a former professor of oral medicine at the University of Alabama, explains why: "Vitamin C in the urine tends to bind calcium and decrease its free form. This means less chance of calcium's separating out as calcium oxalate (stones)."[1] So vitamin C inhibits the union of calcium and oxalate, *reducing* the risk of oxalate kidney stones.

Among the most important risk factors for kidney stones is dehydration, especially among the elderly.[2] Vegetable juicing provides lots of hydration (veggie juice is mostly water). Also, the diuretic effect of vitamin C reduces the urine concentration of oxalate. Fast moving rivers deposit little silt.

Tea and coffee are thought to be the largest sources of oxalate in the diet of many people, accounting for up to 150–300 mg a day.[3,4] This intake is considerably more than would likely be generated by a vitamin C (ascorbate) dose of 1,000 mg a day.[5,6] Ascorbate in low or high doses generally does not cause a significant increase in urinary oxalate.[7–11] Ascorbate tends to *prevent* formation of calcium oxalate kidney stones.[12,13]

Magnesium

Magnesium has an important role in the prevention of kidney stone formation.[14] Magnesium stimulates production of calcitonin, a substance that draws calcium out of the blood and soft tissues, and back into the bones, preventing some forms of arthritis and kidney stones. Magnesium suppresses parathyroid hormone, preventing it from breaking down bone. Magnesium converts vitamin D into its active form so that it can assist in calcium absorption. Magnesium is required to activate an enzyme that is necessary to form new bone. Magnesium regulates active calcium transport. All these factors help place calcium where it needs to be, and not in kidney stones.

One of magnesium's many jobs is to keep calcium in solution to prevent it from solidifying into crystals; even at times of dehydration, if there is sufficient magnesium, calcium will stay in solution. Magnesium is a pivotal treatment for kidney stones. If you don't have enough magnesium to help dissolve calcium, you will end up with various forms of calcification. This translates into kidney stones, muscle spasms, fibrositis, fibromyalgia, and atherosclerosis (as in calcification of the arteries). George Bunce, Ph.D., has clinically demonstrated the relationship between kidney stones and magnesium deficiency. As early as 1964, Bunce reported the benefits of administering a 420 mg dose of magnesium oxide a day to people who had a history of frequent stone formation.[15,16] If poorly absorbed magnesium oxide works, other forms of better-absorbed magnesium will work better.

Calcium oxalate stones can effectively be prevented by getting an adequate amount of magnesium, either through foods high in magnesium (buckwheat, green vegetables, beans, nuts), or magnesium supplements. Take a magnesium supplement with *at least* the U.S. RDA of 300–400 mg a day (more may be desirable in order to maintain an ideal 1:1 balance of magnesium to calcium). To prevent a laxative effect, take a supplement that is readily absorbable, such as magnesium citrate, chelate, malate, or chloride. Magnesium oxide, mentioned above, is cheap and widely available. However, only about 5 percent of magnesium oxide is absorbed; the other 95 percent acts mostly as a laxative.[17] Milk of magnesia (magnesium hydroxide) is even more of a laxative, and unsuitable for supplementation. Magnesium citrate is a good choice; it is easy to find, relatively inexpensive, and well absorbed. Usually 400 mg of supplemental magnesium is adequate.

Oxalate stones can also be prevented by adequate quantities of B-complex vitamins and magnesium. Any common B-complex supplement, twice daily, will suffice.

A Dozen Ways to Reduce Your Risk of Kidney Stones

1. Maximize fluid intake.[18] Especially drink fruit and vegetable juices. Orange, grape, and carrot juices are high in citrates which inhibit a buildup of uric acid and also stop calcium salts from forming.[19]

2. Control urine pH. Slightly acidic urine helps prevent urinary tract infections, dissolves both phosphate and struvite stones, and will not cause calcium oxalate stones. And, of course, one way to make urine slightly acidic is to take vitamin C.

3. Avoid excessive oxalates by not overconsuming rhubarb, spinach, chocolate, or dark tea or coffee.

4. Lose weight. Being overweight is associated with substantially increased risk of kidney stones.[20]

5. Keep tabs on blood pressure. A history of hypertension is a risk factor for kidney stones. Check with your health care provider on this one. Checking your own blood pressure at home once a week is a good idea, too.

6. Do not omit calcium from the diet. Calcium is probably not the real culprit. Low blood calcium levels may actually cause calcium stones.[21] Most kidney stones are compounds of calcium and yet many Americans are calcium deficient. Instead of lowering your calcium intake, reduce excess dietary phosphorus by avoiding carbonated soft drinks, especially colas. Cola soft drinks contain excessive quantities of phosphorus as phosphoric acid. This is the same acid that is used by dentists to dissolve tooth enamel before applying bonding resins.

7. Take a magnesium supplement that provides *at least* the U.S. RDA of 300–400 mg a day. More may be desirable in order to maintain what many practitioners consider to be an ideal 1:1 balance of magnesium to calcium. Many people eating "modern" processed-food diets do not consume optimal quantities of magnesium.

8. Take a good B-complex vitamin supplement, twice daily, that contains pyridoxine (vitamin B_6). A deficiency of vitamin B_6 produces kidney stones in experimental animals. Vitamin B_6 deficiency is very common in humans. A vitamin B_1 (thiamine) deficiency also is associated with kidney stones.[22]

9. To control uric acid stones, which are caused by a problem metabolizing purines and may form in a condition such as gout, stop eating meat. Nutrition tables and textbooks indicate meat as the major dietary purine source. Natural treatments add juice fasts and eating sour cherries. Increased vitamin C consumption helps by improving the urinary excretion of uric acid.[23] For these stones, use buffered ascorbate C.

10. People with cystine stones (only 1 percent of all kidney stones) should follow a low-methionine diet and use buffered vitamin C.

11. Kidney stones are associated with a high sugar intake, so eat less (or no) added sugar.[24]

12. Infections can cause conditions that favor stone formation, such as overly concentrated urine (from fever sweating, vomiting, or diarrhea). Practice good preventive health care, and it will pay you back with interest.

RESOURCES

Education should make you want to learn more.
—Jean Frances Chamberlin Saul (1919–2001)
(Montclair State College, Class of 1941:
our mother and grandmother, respectively)

"Look at all the things we can do without," mused my mother, upon receipt of a new mail-order catalog. Movie complexes have upwards of eight screens, yet it is tough to find one good film. Cable TV: 200 channels and nothing worth watching. With computers, it's GIGO: garbage in, garbage out. You even need intellectual hip boots to wade through the useless volumes that crowd our libraries. Our information superhighway is fast becoming an information landfill, resulting in a lot of people being over-informed and under-educated.

Wisdom is the reduction of a complex jumble of theories down to the simple, effective, economical, and life supporting. We do not know it all, nor do we have the whole story, nor the final answer. The good news is that there are many excellent sources of information about the therapeutic benefits of juicing. Here's a listing, with our comments, of just *some* of the great books, movies, and organizations you can check out. Caution: One good thing leads to another.

RECOMMENDED READING
WITH ANNOTATED BIBLIOGRAPHY

Classics on Juicing and Nutrition

Benjamin, Harry. *Everybody's Guide to Nature Cure.* Hesperides Press, 2008; a rare book originally published in 1936 in London by Health for All Publishing Company. This British naturopath recommended fasting and raw foods and juices for nearly every imaginable condition. At the time I read it (1975) I thought he was off his trolley. Turns out he was right. Of all the books that have set me on the course I am on today, this book is near the top of the list. It was written in 1936. I hope my books are still in print after seventy-five years.

Gregory, Dick. *Dick Gregory's Natural Diet for Folks Who Eat: Cookin' with Mother Nature.* NY: Harper and Row, 1983; originally published 1973. A little humor never hurts an important work. Dick Gregory once weighed nearly 300 pounds. He began fasting and eating only fresh and raw foods and lost well over 100 pounds. But it's what he found in the process that is even more important. Gregory describes how his health problems went away and how much better he and his family now feel on "Mother Nature's" diet. His personal story is of course included, and it is witty and inspiring reading. Also included is the best twenty-one-page introduction to human structure and function that can be found anywhere (see Chapter 4, "The Body Owner's Manual"). The chapter on fasting is enough to get the reader to try it; it certainly worked with me.

Howell, Edward. *Food Enzymes for Health and Longevity.* Woodstock Valley, CT: Omangod Press, 1980; originally published in 1939, without the word "Food" leading the title. Dr. Howell's treatise on raw food enzymes stands as something of a classic in naturopathic healing. His work is documented with over 400 references, which regrettably are not included in this modern paperback reprint. Since all of those references were pre-1940, their inclusion would provide a fine historical review as well as substantiation for Dr. Howell's position. His position is well thought out and carefully presented nonetheless: eat fresh and raw food for at least 75 percent of your diet. This book is a thorough and scholarly work that explains in detail what cooked food can do to the body and what raw food can do for a body. The introduction by raw foods advocate Viktoras Kulvinskas is worth reading and is followed with a recent interview with Dr. Howell. A good summary appears at the close of the book. There are newer editions of this book, which have received mixed reviews. Howell has also written *Enzyme Nutrition* (1995).

Illich, Ivan. *Limits to Medicine: Medical Nemesis, the Expropriation of Health*. London: Marion Boyars Publishers, 2010; originally published in 1975 as *Medical Nemesis: The Expropriation of Health*. A "nemesis" is an enemy; "expropriation" may be defined as the deprivation of rights. In this incredibly well-documented book, Dr. Illich puts forward an ironclad argument that allopathic medicine has turned against us and is literally depriving us of our health. A viewpoint like that will not just "go away" when one chapter alone (The Medicalization of Life) contains 264 foot-notes. Illich speaks of doctors as "medical clergy" and their activities as disease producing, or iatrogenic. This means that the medical monopoly is making us sick. Illich provides solutions as well as enumerating problems, but the author of *Deschooling Society* (1971) has some revolutionary ideas to share. Absolutely vital reading for anyone who contracts his or her health out to a doctor or hospital.

Kulvinskas, Viktoras. *Survival in the 21st Century*. Summertown, TN: Book Publishing Company, 2010; originally published in 1975. Here's a book that is certain to offend almost everybody, and equally certain to educate almost everybody. If the reader can get past the gaudily mod-retro cover and the hippie-ish illustrations, he or she will uncover an unusually well-documented handbook on how to live healthfully and very economically on a raw foods diet. Kulvinskas, a raw foods advocate and co-founder of the Hippocrates Health Institute, makes a convincing argu-ment with the support of 259 citations from a variety of sources. A vast amount of practical information is provided on how and why, with an emphasis on sprouted seeds. Later chapters deal with spiritual discipline and practices that may or may not be embraced by the reader. It is not necessary to accept every word Kulvinskas writes. His case for natural diet is outstanding.

Natural Hygiene Society (of America). *The Greatest Health Discovery.* Chicago: IL. Natural Hygiene Press, Inc., 1972. I would catch a little flak from my doctoral students every time I'd trot out old research studies from the 1940s, 50s, and 60s. Now to *really* annoy them: here's a book of largely pre-Civil War sources of drugless healing. For when hygienists speak of the 40s and 50s, you don't even know at first which century they are referring to. The natural hygiene lifestyle not only avoids drugs, but also involves neither supplements or nor remedies of any kind. Its reliance on clean living, sunshine, water, unprocessed raw food, and therapeutic fasting is straight out of the 1800s.

The Greatest Health Discovery is a condensed recap of the writers and ideas that have shaped some 200 years of an American version of macrobiotics, and is a veritable natural health Hall of Fame. It includes Sylvester Graham (born in 1794), who is known for the coarse whole-grain crackers that bear his name. Did you know that his lecture in my hometown of Rochester, New York, drew 3,000 people at a time when all roads leading to it were made of dirt? (I missed hearing him by just over a hundred years.) There's James Calab Jackson, M.D., abolitionist and founder of what was the world's largest naturopathic hospital in Dansville, New York. There's John H. Tilden, M.D., the originator of the theory of systemic toxemia as the root cause of all illness, and the work of twentieth century author Herbert M. Shelton, N.D., D.C.

A favorite account is that of Russell Thacker Trall, M.D., who founded the first hydrotherapy facility in the United States in 1844, and is credited with setting down a system of natural hygiene still followed to this day. So convinced was Dr. Trall that drugs were poisons and that food and water would cure, that during the Civil War he wrote to various departments in Washington and to President Lincoln himself, offering "a system of the healing art, which, applied to the treatment of the diseases prevailing in the camps and hospitals of our armies, would save thousands of the lives of our officers and soldiers" (pg. 55). Trall's successful patients included members of Congress. When he lectured at the Smithsonian Institution in February 1862, he argued that Willie Lincoln, the President's teenage son, need not have died from "a cold, a pneumonia or a fever" but to no avail. To this day, presidents and Congress are yet to act on the advice of natural healing advocates.

And by the way, Dr. Trall's letters were not answered, either.

Newman, Laura D. *Make Your Juicer Your Drug Store*. CA, Paso Robles: Benedict Lust Publications, 1998; originally published in 1970. A fellow student placed this book in my hands at Andover Newton Theological School in October of 1974. I remember the time, the book, and its impact on me, but not the student's name. Thank you, sir, over the decades.

Walker, Norman W. *The Vegetarian Guide to Diet & Salad*. Norwalk Press, 1995; previously published as *Diet and Salad Suggestions,* 1971. Walker, the grand gentleman of juicing, lived to be ninety-nine years (and five months) old. He made good use of his time, writing a large number of books on juicing and raw foods. Here are some: *Fresh Vegetable and Fruit Juices* (1936); *Become Younger* (1949); *The Natural Way to Vibrant Health* (1972); *Back to the Land for Self Preservation* (1977); *Colon Health Key to Vibrant Life* (1979); *Pure and Simple Natural Weight Control* (1981); and *Raw Vegetable Juices: What's Missing in Your Body* (2003).

Warmbrand, Max. *Encyclopedia of Health and Nutrition*. NY: Pyramid Books, 1962. The author has been largely forgotten but the book has a vast amount of material worth your time. There are some newer editions, but this one remains somewhat difficult to locate.

Wigmore, Ann. *Recipes for Longer Life*. New York: Avery Publishing Group, 1982; originally published in 1978. What makes this book rather unique is that it is a cookbook . . . with absolutely no cooking in it. Ann Wigmore can help you really enjoy a raw foods diet. She was the woman largely responsible for bringing sprouting to the United States and she had decades of experience in helping people get well using raw foods, sprouts, juices, and fasting. It's all here: salads, dressings (over thirty different ones), dips, spreads, sauces, breads, and soups (yes, without cooking), candies, cookies, pies and, of course, entrees. How to sprout, juice, and gradually move toward such a diet is also included.

I met "Dr. Ann" in Buffalo many years ago. She was just as advertised: knowledgeable, gracious, and energetic. She literally put this book into my hands with her good wishes. Dr. Ann is also the author of *Be Your Own Doctor* (1982), *The Hippocrates Diet and Health Program* (1983), *The Wheatgrass Book* (1985), *The Sprouting Book* (1986), *The Blending Book* (1997), and her very captivating autobiography *Why Suffer? How I Overcame Illness & Pain Naturally* (1985).

Other Books and Articles on Juicing

We have been listing some of the classics that have stood the test of time and experience. Here are some newer juicing books that are up-to-date and readily available through any bookseller. Remember, this is just a partial listing. Search the Internet, read reviews, and choose for yourself.

Calbom, Cherie. *The Juice Lady's Guide to Juicing for Health: Unleashing the Healing Power of Whole Fruits and Vegetables.* Revised ed. New York: Avery Publishing Group, 2008.

_____. *The Juice Lady's Turbo Diet: Lose Ten Pounds in Ten Days—the Healthy Way!* Lake Mercy, FL: Siloam, 2010.

_____. *Juicing, Fasting, and Detoxing for Life: Unleash the Healing Power of Fresh Juices and Cleansing Diets.* New York: Grand Central Life & Style (2008).

Crocker, Pat. *The Juicing Bible.* 2nd ed. Toronto: Robert Rose, 2008.

David, E.L. "The Red Beetroot Juice." *Let's Live* March 1962: 7, 55.

Jacobs, Carole. *The Everything Juicing Book: All You Need to Create Delicious Juices for your Optimum Health.* Avon, MA: Adams Media, 2010.

Manheim, Jason. *The Healthy Green Drink Diet: Advice and Recipes to Energize, Alkalize, Lose Weight, and Feel Great.* New York: Skyhorse Publishing, 2012.

Murray, Michael. *Complete Book of Juicing: Your Delicious Guide to Youthful Vitality.* New York: Clarkson Potter, 1997.

Owen, Sarah. *The Top 100 Juices: 100 Juices to Turbo-Charge Your Body with Vitamins and Minerals.* London: Duncan Baird Publishers, 2007.

Savona, Natalie. *The Big Book of Juices: More Than 400 Natural Blends for Health and Vitality Every Day.* London: Duncan Baird Publishers, 2010.

Shazzie. *Detox Your World.* Reprint ed. Berkeley, CA: North Atlantic Books, 2012.

Wood, Rebecca. *The New Whole Foods Encyclopedia: A Comprehensive Resource for Healthy Eating.* Revised ed. New York: Penguin Books, 1999.

Books on the Gerson Therapy

Gerson, Max. *A Cancer Therapy: Results of Fifty Cases*. 3rd ed. Carmel, CA: Totality Books, 1977. Dr. Gerson had striking success in frequently curing cancer, circulatory and nervous diseases, tuberculosis, arthritis, and more. His book completely describes the details of the Gerson therapy, thereby taking the wind out of the sails of those who would say that Gerson was, and his institute is, out for financial gain. Unlike some books that tell of a cure, this one tells exactly how to cure. Pages 187 to 248 should be read first by anyone who needs immediate knowledge of the therapy. Pages 251 to 389 contain the fifty case histories, including x-rays, of those cured of a considerable variety of cancers. Gerson explains his approach, and the problem of cancer in general, in the first third of the book. Gerson's therapy can be done at home with minimal professional care. Here is far more than just "hope" for incurable illness; here is a proven solution. You probably do not believe that statement. That is why you need to read this book.

Straus, Howard. *Dr. Max Gerson: Healing the Hopeless*. 2nd ed. Carmel, CA: Totality Books, 2009. This is the definitive biography of Max Gerson, M.D., written by his grandson. I know the author personally, and he is a tall, muscular, vibrant fellow . . . and very vegetarian. If there were ever a walking argument for Dr. Gerson's work, he is it. To read a review of the book, go to http://www.doctoryourself.com/ gersonbio.htm.

More Books on the Gerson Therapy

Gerson, Charlotte, Straus H, Gerson M. *The Gerson Primer: Practical Guidance, Resources and Recipes for Gerson Therapy Patients*. 4th ed. Bonita, CA: Gerson Institute, 1996.

Gerson Charlotte. Walker M. Reprint ed. *The Gerson Therapy: The Amazing Nutritional Therapy for Cancer and Other Illnesses*. New York: Kensington Publishing Corp., 2006.

Haught, S.J. *Censured for Curing Cancer: The American Experience of Dr. Max Gerson*. 2nd ed. Barrytown, NY: Station Hill Press, 1991.

Gerson Charlotte. *Defeating Arthritis, Bone and Joint Diseases*. Carmel, CA: Gerson Health Media, 2011.

_____. *Defeating Obesity, Diabetes and High Blood Pressure: The Metabolic Syndrome*. Carmel, CA: Gerson Health Media, 2010.

_____. *Healing the Gerson Way: Defeating Cancer and Other Chronic Diseases*. 2nd ed. Carmel, CA: Totality Books, 2009. Reviewed at http://orthomolecular.org/library/jom/2007/pdf/2007-v22n04-p217.pdf.

RECOMMENDED MOVIES ON JUICING AND MORE

Banzhaf, John. *Super Size Me*. DVD. Directed by Morgan Spurlock. Culver City, CA: Sony Pictures Entertainment, 2004.

Cross, Joe. *Fat, Sick, and Nearly Dead*. DVD. Directed by Joe Cross. Warren, NJ: Passion River Films, 2010.

Gerson, Charlotte. *The Gerson Miracle*. DVD. Directed by Steve Kroschel. Los Angeles: Cinema Libre, 2009.

Kroschel, Garrett. *The Beautiful Truth*. DVD. Directed by Garrett Kroschel. Los Angeles: Cinema Libre, 2008.

Kroschel, Steve. *Dying to Have Known*. DVD. Directed by Steve Kroschel. Los Angeles: Cinema Libre, 2006.

Saul, Andrew. *Food Matters*. DVD. Directed by James Colquhoun. Warren, NJ: Passion River Films, 2008.

ONLINE RESOURCES

Health and Nutrition

Doctor Yourself.com. A complete listing of Andrew W. Saul's 180 publications is at http://www.doctoryourself.com/publications.html.

Feingold Association of the United States. The organization states: "Numerous studies show that certain synthetic food additives can have serious learning, behavior, and/or health effects for sensitive people." Learn what to do at http://www.feingold.org/research.php and http://www.feingold .org/newsletters.php; free email newsletter available at http://www.fein gold.org/ON.html.

Living and Raw Foods. http://www.rawfoods.com provides literally hundreds of raw food/natural hygiene links.

Price-Pottenger Nutrition Foundation.The nutrition research of Francis Pottenger, M.D. (and that of Weston Price, D.D.S.) can be found at http://www.price-pottenger.org.

"Raising Student Achievement through Better Nutrition" by Helen Saul Case is available for free access at http://orthomolecular.org/library/jom/2006/pdf/2006-v21n02-p79.pdf.

Vegetarianism. There are doctors supportive of vegetarianism, and here they are: The Physicians' Committee for Responsible Medicine at http://www.pcrm.org; free download of their "New Four Food Groups" at http://www.pcrm.org/health/veginfo/vsk/4foodgroups.pdf.

Organic Gardening and Farming

Soil and Health Library. http://www.soilandhealth.org is a free, online library of organic gardening, natural farming, and nutrition; many obscure, hard-to-find books freely available. Highly recommended.

Orthomolecular (Nutritional) Medicine

Gerson Institute. http://www.gerson.org.

Journal of Orthomolecular Medicine (*JOM*) Online Archive. Nearly forty-five years of *JOM* are available as full-text pdf downloads, free of charge at http://orthomolecular.org/library/jom/index.shtml.

Orthomolecular Medicine News Service Online Archive. Online access to nearly 100 issues at

http://orthomolecular.org/resources/omns/index.shtml.

Practitioner Directories. To locate a physician near you who uses orthomolecular medicine, go to http://orthomolecular.org/resources/omns/v06n09.shtml.

References

Chapter 1: Confessions of the Dad Who Made His Kids Drink Vegetable Juices

1. Shaw, G.B. *The Vegetarian* (January 15, 1898).

2. Pacini, A.J. "Why We Need Vitamin E." *Health Culture* Magazine (January 1936).

3. Bacharach A.L. "Vitamin E and Habitual Abortion." *Brit Med J* i (1940): 890 (cited in *The Vitamins in Medicine* by F. Bicknell and F. Prescott. Milwaukee: Lee Foundation for Nutritional Research, 1953: 632.

4. Semba, R.D. "Vitamin A, Immunity, and Infection." *Clin Infect Dis* 19(3) (September 1994): 489–499; Werbach, M.R., J. Moss. *Textbook of Nutritional Medicine*. Tarzana, CA: Third Line Press, 1999.

5. Saul, A.W. *Doctor Yourself: Natural Healing That Works*. Laguna Beach, CA: Basic Health Publications, 2003.

6. Diplock, A.T. "Safety of Antioxidant Vitamins and Beta-Carotene." *Am J Clin Nutr* 62(6) (1995): 1510S–1516S; Bendich, A. "The Safety of Beta-Carotene." *Nutr-Cancer* 11(4) (1988): 207–214.

7. Case, H.S. *The Vitamin Cure for Women's Health Problems*. Laguna Beach, CA: Basic Health Publications, 2012.

Chapter 4: Health Benefits from Juicing

1. Cheney, G. "Vitamin U Therapy of Peptic Ulcer." *Calif Med* 77(4) (October 1952): 248–252. Vitamin U was the provisional name Dr. Cheney gave to the unknown factor(s) in cabbage that heal ulcers. These substances are yet to be fully explored, but almost certainly include vitamin C, glutamine, glucosinolates, and ascorbigen, also known as cabbagen. See also: Cheney, G., H Waxler, I.J. Miller. "Vitamin U Therapy of Peptic Ulcer: Experience at San Quentin Prison." *Calif Med* 84(1) (January 1956): 39–42; Cheney, G. "The Medical Management of Gastric Ulcers with Vitamin U Therapy." *Stanford Med Bull* 13(2) (May 1955: 204–214; Cheney, G. "Vitamin U Concentrate Therapy of Peptic Ulcer." *Am J Gastroenterol* 21(3) (March 1954): 230–250; Cheney, G. "Anti-Peptic Ulcer Dietary Factor

(Vitamin "U") in the Treatment of Peptic Ulcer." *J Am Diet Assoc* 26(9) (September 1950): 668–672; Cheney, G. The Nature of the Antipepticulcer Dietary Factor. *Stanford Med Bull* 8(3) (August 1950): 144–161.

2. *JAMA* 163:14, (April 6, 1957): 1311.

3. Saul, A. *Fire Your Doctor! How to Be Independently Healthy.* Laguna Beach, CA: Basic Health Publications, 2005.

4. Zeratsky, K. *Mayo Clinic Online.* "Vegetable Juice: As Good as Whole Vegetables?" Available at www.mayoclinic.com/health/vegetable-juice/AN01857 (accessed April 21, 2012).

5. Gebhardt, S.E., R.G. Thomas. "Vitamin A." Nutritive Value of Foods. U.S. Department of Agriculture, Agricultural Research Service, Home and Garden Bulletin 72 (2002). Available at http://www.nal.usda.gov/fnic/foodcomp/Data/HG72/hg72_2002.pdf.

6. U.S. Department of Agriculture. Center for Nutrition Policy and Promotion. "Report of the Dietary Guidelines Advisory Committee on the Dietary Guidelines for Americans, 2010. Part B. Section 2: The Total Diet: Combining Nutrients, Consuming Food." Available at http://www.cnpp.usda.gov/Publications/Dietary Guidelines/2010/DGAC/ Report/B-2-TotalDiet.pdf (accessed November 2011).

7. Centers for Disease Control and Prevention. Nutrition for Everyone. "How Many Fruits and Vegetables Do You Need?" Available at http://www.fruitsandveggiesmatter .gov/downloads/General_Audience_Brochure.pdf (accessed November 2011).

8. Centers for Disease Control and Prevention. CDC Online Newsroom. "Majority of Americans Not Meeting Recommendations for Fruit and Vegetable Consumption." Press Release, September 29, 2009. Available at http://www.cdc.gov/media/pressrel/2009/r090929.htm (accessed November 2011).

9. Casagrande, S.S., Y. Wang, C. Anderson, et al. "Have Americans Increased Their Fruit and Vegetable Intake? The Trends between 1988 and 2002." *Am J Prev Med* 32:4 (April 2007): 257–263. Available at http://www.fruitsandveggiesmorematters.org/wp-content/uploads/UserFiles/File/pdf/press/AJPM_32–4_Casagrande_with%20embargo.pdf (accessed November 2011).

10. Balch, J.F., P.A. Balch. *Prescriptions for Natural Healing.* New York: Avery Publishing Group, 1990.

11. U. S. Department of Agriculture. "USDA and HHS Announce New Dietary Guidelines to Help Americans Make Healthier Food Choices and Confront Obesity Epidemic." Press Release, January 11, 2011. Available at http://www.cnpp.usda.gov/Publications/Dietary Guidelines/2010/PolicyDoc/PressRelease.pdf. (accessed November 2011).

12. Gandini, S., H. Merzenich, C. Robertson, et al. "Meta-Analysis of Studies on Breast Cancer Risk and Diet: The Role of Fruit and Vegetable Consumption and the Intake of Associated Micronutrients." *Eur J Cancer* 36:5 (March 2000): 636–646. Riboli, E., T. Norat. "Epidemiologic Evidence of the Protective Effect of Fruit and Vegetables on Cancer Risk." *Am J Clin Nutr* 78:(3 Suppl) (September 2003): 559S–569S. U.S. Department of Agriculture. Center for Nutrition, Policy, and Promotion. "Report of the Dietary Guidelines Advisory Committee on the Dietary Guidelines for Americans, 2010. Part D. Section 5:

Carbohydrates." Table D4.2. Available at http://www.cnpp.usda.gov/Publications/ DietaryGuidelines/2010/DGAC/Report/D-5-Carbohydrates.pdf (accessed November 2011). McCann, S.E., J.L. Freudenheim, J.R. Marshall, et al. "Risk of Human Ovarian Cancer Is Related to Dietary Intake of Selected Nutrients, Phytochemicals and Food Groups." *J Nutr* 133:6 (June 2003):1937–1942.

13. Liu, S., J.E. Manson, I.M. Lee, et al. "Fruit and Vegetable Intake and Risk of Cardiovascular Disease: The Women's Health Study." *Am J Clin Nutr* 72:4 (October 2000): 922–928. Hung, H.C., K.J. Joshipura, R. Jiang, et al. "Fruit and Vegetable Intake and Risk of Major Chronic Disease." *J Natl Cancer Inst* 96:21 (2004): 1577–1584.

14. Block, G., B. Patterson, A. Subar. "Fruit, Vegetables, and Cancer Prevention: A Review of the Epidemiological Evidence." *Nutr Cancer* 18:1 (1992): 1–29.

15. Blanchard, C.M., K.S. Courneya, K. Stein. "Cancer Survivors' Adherence to Lifestyle Behavior Recommendations and Associations with Health-Related Quality of Life: Results from the American Cancer Society's SCS-II." *J Clin Oncol* 26:13 (May 1, 2008): 2198–2204.

16. Reed, J., E. Frazão, R. Itskowitz. U.S. Department of Agriculture. Economic Research Service. "How Much Do Americans Pay for Fruits and Vegetables?" Agriculture Information Bulletin, October 2004. Available at http://www.ers.usda.gov/publications/aib792/ aib792-4/aib792-4.pdf (accessed November 2011).

17. Ibid.

18. U.S. Department of Agriculture. Economic Research Service. "Access to Affordable and Nutritious Food: Measuring and Understanding Food Deserts and Their Consequences." Report to Congress (June 2009). Available at http://www.ers.usda.gov/Publications/AP/ AP036/AP036.pdf. (accessed November 2011).

19. Ibid.

20. Alexander, M., et al: "Oral Beta-carotene Can Increase the Number of OKT4 Cells in Human Blood." *Immunology Letters* 9 (1985): 221–224.

21. Tang, A.M., N. Graham, A.J. Kirby, et al. "Dietary Micronutrient Intake and Risk of Progression to Acquired Immunodeficiency Syndrome (AIDS) in Human Immunodeficiency Virus Type 1 (HIV-1) Infected Homosexual Men." *Am J Epidemiol* 138(11) (December 1993): 937–951.

22. Merck. *Merck Manual* 14th ed. West Point, PA: Merck & Company, 1982, 891.

23. Ibid.

24. Potter, A.S., S. Foroudi, A. Stamatikos, et al. "Drinking Carrot Juice Increases Total Antioxidant Status and Decreases Lipid Peroxidation in Adults." *Nutr J* 10 (September 24, 2011): 96.

25. Jansen, R.J., D.P. Robinson, R.Z. Stolzenberg-Solomon, et al. "Fruit and Vegetable Consumption Is Inversely Associated with Having Pancreatic Cancer." *Cancer Causes Control* 22 (September 14, 2011): 1613–1625.

26. Zaini, R., M.R. Clench, C.L. Le Maitre. "Bioactive Chemicals from Carrot (*Daucus*

carota) Juice Extracts for the Treatment of Leukemia." *J Med Food* 14 (August 24, 2011): 1303-1312.

27. Culbert, M. *ICHF* Magazine 7:2 (Fall 2004). Available at http://www.ichf.info/history.php.

28. Blanchard, C.M., K.S. Courney, K. Stein. "Cancer Survivors' Adherence to Lifestyle Behavior Recommendations and Associations with Health-Related Quality of Life: Results from the American Cancer Society's SCS-II." *J Clin Oncol* 26:13 (May 2008): 2198–2204.

29. Read, J.A., S.B. Choy, P. Beale P, et al. "An Evaluation of the Prevalence of Malnutrition in Cancer Patients Attending the Outpatient Oncology Clinic. *Asia-Pacific Journal of Clinical Oncology* 2:2 (May 10, 2006): 80–86. Available at http://onlinelibrary.wiley.com/doi/10.1111/j.1743-7563.2006.00048.x/abstract.

30. Bircher, R. "A Turning Point in Nutritional Science." Reprint No. 80. Milwaukee, WI: Lee Foundation for Nutritional Research, 7–8.

Chapter 5: Mega-Nutrition from Vegetables

1. Sirisha, K. "In vitro Anticancer Activity of Betanin, Fresh Juice and Hydro-alcoholic Root Extract of *Beta Vulgaris* on HL-60 Cell Lines." Master's in Pharmacy Dissertation Protocol, Rajiv Gandhi University of Health Sciences, Karnataka, Bangalore (2010–2012): 2–10.

2. Nottingham, S. "Beetroot: Health and Nutrition." Chapter 6. (2004): 1–17, http://www.stephennottingham.co.uk/beetroot6.htm; Lee C.H., M. Wettasinghe, B.W. Bolling, et al. "Betalains: Phase II Enzyme-Inducing Components from Red Beetroot (*Beta vulgaris L.*) Extracts." *Nutr Cancer* 53:1 (2005): 91–103; "*Beta vulgaris:* The Common Beet." USDA Plant Profile. Available at http://plants.usda.gov/java/profile?symbol=BEVU2; Kujala T., J. Loponen, K. Pihlaja. "Betalains and Phenolics in Red Beetroot (*Beta Vulgaris*) Peel Extracts: Extraction and Characterisation." *Z Naturforsch C* 56 (May–June 2001): 343–348; Sturzoiu A., M. Stroescu, A. Stoica, et al. "Betanine Extraction from *Beta Vulgaris* Experimental Research and Statistical Modeling." *U.P.B. Sci Bull* 73:1 (2011): 145–156; Winkler, C., B. Wirleitner, K. Schroecksnadel, et al. "In vitro Effects of Beet Root Juice on Stimulated and Unstimulated Peripheral Blood Mononuclear Cells." *Am J Biochem Biotech* 1:4 (2005): 180–185; Edenharder, R., P. Kurz, K. John, et al. "In vitro Effect of Vegetable and Fruit Juices on the Mutagenicity of 2-Amino-3-Methylimidazole[4,5-F]Quinoline, 2,Amino,3,8-Dimethylimide-3-ol[4,5f]Quinoxaline." *Food Chem Toxicol* 32 (1994): 443–459; Kapadia, G.J., H. Tokudab, T. Konoshimac, te al. "Chemoprevention of Lung and Skin Cancer by *Beta Vulgaris* (Beet) Root Extract." *Cancer Lett* 100 (1996): 211-214; Eastwood, M.A., H. Nyhlin. "Beeturia and Colonic Oxalic Acid. *QJM* 88:10 (1995): 711–717; see also: Neelwarne, B., ed. *Red Beet Biotechnology: Food and Pharmaceutical Applications.* New York: Springer, 2012.

3. Ferenczi, A. "Tumor Treatment with Red Beets and Anthocyans, Respectively." *Zeitschrift Fuer die Gesamte Innere Medizin und Ihire Grenzgebiete* 16 (1961): 180. Available at http://www.docstoc.com/docs/31941644/Tumor-Treatment-with-Red-Beets-and-Anthocyans_-respectively.

4. Martinotti, M. "Just Beet It. Formerly Known as a Health Supplement, Betaine Is Gain-

ing Some Real Muscle." *Muscle and Performance*. Available at http://www.muscleand performancemag.com/nutrition-supplements/2012/1/just-beet-it (accessed Dec 2012).

5. González, M.J., J.R. Miranda-Massari, A.W. Saul. *I Have Cancer: What Should I Do?* Laguna Beach, CA: Basic Health Publishers, 2009.

6. Christen, A.G., J.A. Christen. "Horace Fletcher (1849-1919): The Great Masticator." *J Hist Dent* 45:3 (November 1997): 95–100.

7. McCabe, P. "Naturopathy, Nightingale, and Nature Cure: A Convergence of Interests." *Complement Ther Nurs Midwifery* 6:1 (February 2000): 4–8.

Appendix 2: Interview of Andrew W. Saul by Nancy Desjardins

1. Morgan, G., R. Ward, M. Barton. *Clinical Oncology* 16 (2004): 549–560.

Appendix 3: Another *Reader's Digest* Absurdity

1. Woolston, C. "Is Meat Good or Bad for You?" *Reader's Digest* (July/August 2012): 36–38.

2. Pan A., Q. Sun, A.M. Bernstein, et al. "Red Meat Consumption and Mortality: Results from Two Prospective Cohort Studies." *Arch Intern Med* 172:7 (2012): 555–563.

3. Woolsten. "Is Meat Good or Bad for You?": 36–38.

4. Ibid.

5. Putnam, J., J. Allshouse, L.S. Kantor. "U.S. Per Capita Food Supply Trends: More Calories, Refined Carbohydrates, and Fats." *Food Review* 25:3 (2002): 2–15. Available at http://ers.usda.gov/publications/FoodReview/DEC2002/frvol25i3a.pdf.

6. Centers for Disease Control and Prevention. CDC Online Newsroom. "Majority of Americans Not Meeting Recommendations for Fruit and Vegetable Consumption." Press release (September 29, 2009). Available at http://www.cdc.gov/media/pressrel/2009/r090929.htm.

7. Casagrande, S.S., Y. Wang, C. Anderson, et al. "Have Americans Increased Their Fruit and Vegetable Intake? The Trends between 1988 and 2002. *Am J Prev Med* 32:4 (April 2007): 257–263. Available at http://www.ajpmonline.org/article/S0749-3797%2806%2900551-4/abstract.

8. Balch, J.F., P.A. Balch. *Prescriptions for Natural Healing*. New York: Avery Publishing Group, 1990.

9. U.S. Department of Agriculture. "USDA Nutrient Database, SR24." (September 28, 2012). Available at http://www.ars.usda.gov/Services/docs.htm?docid=22114.

10. Ibid.

Appendix 4: Preventing Oxalate Kidney Stones

1. Cheraskin, E., M. Ringsdorf Jr, E. Sisley. *The Vitamin C Connection*. New York: Bantam Books, 1983.

2. Manz, F., A. Wentz. "The Importance of Good Hydration for the Prevention of Chronic Diseases." *Nutr Rev* 63: 6 (Pt 2) (2005): S2–S5.

3. Noonan, S.C., G.P. Savage. "Oxalate Content of Foods and Its Effect on Humans." *Asia Pac J Clin Nutr* 8 (1999): 64–74.

4. Gasinska, A., D. Gajewska. "Tea and Coffee as the Main Sources of Oxalate in Diets of Patients with Kidney Oxalate Stones." *Roczn Pzh* 58:1 (2007): 61–67.

5. Robitaille, L., O.A. Mamer OA, W.H. Miller, et al. "Oxalic Acid Excretion after Intravenous Ascorbic Acid Administration." *Metabolism* 58:2 (February 2009): 263–269.

6. Pauling, L. *How to Live Longer And Feel Better.* Corvallis, OR: OSU Press, 2006.

7. Wandzilak, T.R., S.D. D'Andre, P.A. Davis, et al. (1994) "Effect of High Dose Vitamin C on Urinary Oxalate Levels." *J Urology* 151 (1994): 834–837.

8. Hickey, S., A.W. Saul. *Vitamin C: The Real Story, the Remarkable and Controversial Healing Factor.* Laguna Beach, CA: Basic Health Publications, 2008.

9. Hickey, S., H. Roberts. "Vitamin C Does Not Cause Kidney Stones." *OMNS* (July 5, 2005). Available http://orthomolecular.org/resources/omns/v01n07.shtml.

10. Padayatty, S.J., A.Y. Sun, Q. Chen, et al. (2010) "Vitamin C: Intravenous Use by Complementary and Alternative Medicine Practitioners and Adverse Effects." *PLoS One* 5:7 (2010): e11414.

11. See citation 5 above.

12. See citation 8 above.

13. See citation 9 above.

14. Dean C. *The Magnesium Miracle.* New York: Ballantine Books, 2007.

15. Ibid.

16. Bunce, G.E., B.W. Li, N.O. Price, et al. Distribution of Calcium and Magnesium in Rat Kidney Homogenate Fractions Accompanying Magnesium Deficiency Induced Nephrocalcinosis." *Exp Mol Pathol* 21:1 (1974): 16–28.

17. See citation 14 above.

18. See citation 2 above.

19. Carper, J. "Orange Juice May Prevent Kidney Stones." *Intelligencer-Journal* (Lancaster, PA), Jan 5, 1994.

20. Bagga, H.S., T. Chi, J. Miller J, et al. (2013) "New Insights into the Pathogenesis of Renal Calculi. *Urol Clin North Am* 40:1 (February 2013): 1–12.

21. Smith, L.H., et al. "Medical Evaluation of Urolithiasis." *Urol Clin N Am.* 1:2 (1974): 241–260.

22. Hagler, L., R.H. Herman. Oxalate Metabolism, II. *Am J Clin Nutr* 26:8 (1973): 882–889.

23. See citation 6 above.

24. J.A. Thom, et al. "The Influence of Refined Carbohydrate on Urinary Calcium Excretion." *Brit J Urol* 50:7 (1978): 459–464.

INDEX

ABOUT THE AUTHORS

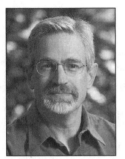

Andrew W. Saul, Ph.D., was known as "The Juicer" when he taught clinical nutrition at New York Chiropractic College and postgraduate continuing education programs. He was also on the faculty of the State University of New York for nine years. Two of those years were spent teaching for the University in both women's and men's penitentiaries (no, not as an inmate). He also taught every grade there is in the Rochester-area parochial and public schools. Dr. Saul is the author or coauthor of eleven books, including *Doctor Yourself: Natural Healing that Works* (Basic Health, 2003) and *Fire Your Doctor!* (Basic Health, 2005). He has published over 180 papers in peer-reviewed publications. Dr. Saul is internationally known for his website www.doctoryourself.com and his appearance in the 2008 documentary movie *Food Matters*.

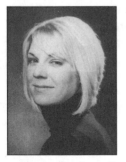

Helen Saul Case, daughter of Andrew W. Saul, is the author of *The Vitamin Cure for Women's Health Problems* (Basic Health, 2012) and has published in the *Journal of Orthomolecular Medicine*. She graduated magna cum laude from Colgate University and then earned a master's degree in education from the State University of New York. She taught English for nine years, is a certified administrator, and worked as English department chair for four years. She currently lives and juices vegetables with her husband and daughter in western New York.